Mindfulness for Women; Mindfulness for Everyone

Harness the Resilient Power of Emotional Balance, Self-Awareness and Living in the Moment to Calm the Chaos Inside

Nicholas Bright

used for personal use. Furthermore, it should not be shared with any other individual or persons for any purpose other than that for which it was initially intended. It is strictly prohibited to amend, reproduce, distribute, utilize, quote, or paraphrase any part of the content within this publication without prior authorization from the writer or publisher. Any violation of these regulations may result in legal action against those who have breached them.

Disclaimer Notice

The presented work is strictly informational and should not be interpreted as an offer to buy or sell any form of security, instrument, or investment vehicle. Furthermore, the information contained herein should not be taken as a medical, legal, tax, accounting, or investment recommendation given by the author(s) or any affiliated company, employees, or paid contributors. In other words, the information is presented without considering individual preferences for specific investments in terms of risk parameters. It is general information that does not account for a person's lifestyle and financial objectives. It is important to note that no tailored advice will be provided based on the given information.

Table of Contents

Welcome to the

Ideas Worth Sharing

Series

My name is Nicholas Bright, and I've spent nearly two decades working as a psychologist specializing in Behavioral Neuroscience and Interpersonal Communication in the US, UK, and Australia. Throughout my career, I've encountered countless stories, experiences, and insights that have shaped my understanding of the human mind and interpersonal interactions.

This series is a collaborative effort, bringing together the experience and expertise of myself and my colleagues: Erica May, Jeff Sharpe, Camila Alvarez, and potentially new faces in the future! We've chosen to write under pen names to respect everyone's privacy and keep the spotlight on the valuable content we offer rather than us as individuals. This decision allows us to freely share our knowledge without the distractions that often come with the limelight. We stand by the authenticity and credibility of the content shared here—our professional integrity remains at the forefront of this series.

We are deeply passionate about our field, and our primary goal is to equip you with practical, research-backed insights that you can implement in your everyday life. Each chapter is designed to inspire and help you better understand yourself and those around you.

We invite you to engage actively with the material: take notes, discuss the ideas with friends and family, and, most importantly, apply the lessons in your daily routine.

1. **Read;** understand what can be done to improve
2. **Reflect;** appreciate your feelings and their origins
3. **Remember;** put your learning into action

Thank you for embarking on this journey of knowledge and growth with us,

Nick

Want to Win Free Books?

Join Our Newsletter!

In this series, we appreciate that someone may find many different books helpful. I certainly know that when discussing sensitive topics like, for example, divorce, we can end up working on grief, anxiety, self-confidence, cognitive dissonance, and lots more. When we encounter a major challenge in life, it is rarely due to one small problem but rather a concoction of our experiences, outlooks, and actions; it's often a deep-rooted issue with many different things we need to uncover and support. We are complicated beings, and we must recognize this. As such, I would love to invite you all to join our newsletter.

In this, I aim to write articles of interest, including excerpts from various books in the series, as well as **vouchers**, **discounts**, and **giveaways**—and of course, no gimmicks or catches. I harbor a deep loathing of companies that offer seemingly amazing deals, only to charge you vast amounts in hidden fees! I vowed to never fall into that trap myself, and any offers I make are designed to be of true benefit and help. If you win a book in a giveaway, I want you to read it with a smile.

Join our newsletter and discover the additional value we can add to your life's curriculum!

Join us at: **www.IdeasWorthSharingSeries.com/newsletter**

See you on the inside!

About the Author: Dr. Nicholas Bright

Dr Nicholas Bright, a highly esteemed Clinical Psychologist based in the vibrant city of New York, is devoted to preventing and treating mental health problems. Nicholas earned his Clinical Psychology degree from Syracuse University, nestled in the heart of New York State. His practice is centred around mindfulness-based therapies, humanistic approaches, and positive psychology principles, enabling individuals to discover their potential and build emotional and psychological resilience.

He has maintained professional ties and a personal friendship with Erica May since their university years. Together, in the Ideas Worth Sharing series, they aim to extend their therapeutic expertise beyond their clinical settings through a series of books on critical psychological topics. This series will delve into various mental health themes, offering comprehensive advice on integrating emotional balance and humanistic practices into everyday life and techniques for fostering positive mental health.

By sharing practical examples and insights from his clinical work, Nick intends to make evidence-based psychological concepts accessible to the general public. His ultimate goal is to empower individuals with the knowledge and tools to manage their mental health effectively, enhance overall well-being, and build resilience.

Preface

"In the midst of movement and chaos,

keep stillness inside of you."

Deepak Chopra

Navigating Life's Storms: A Guide to Mindfulness

At the heart of this guide lies the transformative power of mindfulness, a simple yet profound tool for altering the landscape of your daily life. This book is designed to help you navigate the storms of modern existence without losing sight of what truly matters: your peace, joy, and inner strength. Here, you'll find not only the principles of mindfulness laid out in a clear, accessible manner but also practical strategies for weaving this ancient wisdom into the fabric of your busy life.

I was compelled to write this book after witnessing countless stories of women, much like yourself, who felt overwhelmed by the relentless demands of their careers, families, and personal aspirations. One such story is that of Sarah, a dedicated nurse and mother of three, who was on the brink of burnout. Despite her love for her profession and family, the weight of her responsibilities left her feeling perpetually drained and disconnected. Sarah rediscovered her vitality and joy by integrating mindfulness into her daily routine. Her transformation is one of many that inspired me to share these tools with a broader audience.

The genesis of this book was also heavily influenced by my journey and the profound impact mindfulness has had on my life. Coupled with insights from renowned psychologists and mindfulness practitioners and the real-life experiences of many women during my workshops, this guide was crafted to be your companion in finding serenity amid chaos.

Your support has been invaluable to everyone who has been a part of this journey—collaborators, mentors, family, and friends. Your stories and insights have enriched this guide and deepened my understanding and compassion for those we aim to help.

Thank you, the reader, for choosing to embark on this journey with me. By turning these pages, you are taking a significant step towards reclaiming your mental space and cultivating a more peaceful and fulfilling life. This book is tailored for women between the ages of 25 and 50 who strive to balance multiple roles while seeking sustainable ways to manage stress and enhance their well-being.

As you delve into the following chapters, I invite you to engage actively with the exercises and reflect deeply on how they resonate with your personal experiences. Remember, mindfulness is not merely about reducing stress or enhancing productivity; it is about awakening to your life's potential—here and now.

Thank you once again for your trust and openness. May you find profound wisdom within these pages that light your path to joy and tranquility. I encourage you to read on, apply what resonates with you, and witness the beautiful transformation that awaits.

Introduction

"The present moment is the only time over which we have dominion."

Thich Nhat Hanh

The quest for serenity and joy has never been more critical in our fast-paced world. Amidst the hustle and bustle of daily life, finding a sanctuary of peace within ourselves is an endeavor that resonates with many. This book invites readers on a profound and enlightening journey, exploring the timeless practice of mindfulness as a vehicle for personal transformation and well-being.

The essence of mindfulness is beautifully simple yet deeply profound. It is about being fully present in the moment, aware of our thoughts, emotions, and surroundings, without immediate judgment or reaction. This seemingly straightforward concept is critical to unlocking a more peaceful, joyous, and meaningful existence. The following pages are dedicated to unraveling the layers of mindfulness, illustrating its principles through practical strategies accessible to all.

From the very first chapter, the book elucidates the foundational aspects of mindfulness, establishing a solid understanding upon which readers can begin to build their practice. It demystifies the practice, making it relatable and achievable, and dispels common misconceptions that often deter people from pursuing this path. Through engaging narratives and real-life examples, the book offers a vivid depiction of how mindfulness can be woven into the fabric of daily life.

The progression through the book mirrors the gradual deepening of mindfulness practice itself. Readers are guided through various techniques and exercises, each designed to cultivate a specific aspect of mindfulness. From mindful breathing and meditation to the art of acceptance and letting go, the strategies presented are varied and versatile, catering to each individual's unique needs and circumstances.

Importantly, this book acknowledges the challenges and obstacles that can arise on the path to mindfulness. Rather than portraying these as failures, it reframes them as opportunities for growth and learning. Readers are encouraged to approach their practice with compassion and patience, recognizing that the journey is as significant as the destination.

Integrating mindfulness into one's daily routine is a central theme, with the book offering countless suggestions on how to do so. It emphasizes the practicality of mindfulness, highlighting its relevance and applicability across different spheres of life, including work, relationships, and personal development. This pragmatic approach ensures that the insights gained are theoretical and can lead to tangible improvements in one's quality of life.

Beyond personal peace and joy, the book explores the broader implications of mindfulness on societal well-being. It suggests that individual transformation can ripple outwards, influencing our interactions with others and the planet. Thus, mindfulness is presented as a tool for personal change and a powerful agent for social and environmental harmony.

Throughout these pages, I invite readers to continue their mindfulness practice beyond the book's pages. It positions mindfulness as a lifelong companion rather than a finite goal, encouraging ongoing curiosity, exploration, and growth. The narrative closes with inspirational reflections on mindfulness's profound impact on our lives and the world.

This book is an invitation to embark on a life-changing path towards greater peace, joy, and fulfillment. It stands as a testament to the transformative power of mindfulness, offering guidance, support, and inspiration to all who seek to find calm in the chaos of their daily lives. Through its pages, readers are empowered to cultivate a more profound sense of presence and purpose, navigating the complexities of life with grace and resilience.

Chapter 1: Awakening to Mindfulness

"Mindfulness isn't difficult, we just need

to remember to do it."

Sharon Salzberg

Is Your Mind Full or Are You Mindful?

Finding tranquility can seem like an elusive quest in a world that moves at breakneck speed. Yet, mindfulness offers a sanctuary from the storm—a gentle reminder to anchor ourselves in the present moment. As we embark on this journey together through the initial chapter of our exploration into mindfulness, it is crucial to lay a solid foundation of understanding what mindfulness entails, its profound benefits, and the diverse techniques available to integrate it into our daily lives.

Mindfulness is more than just a buzzword; it's a transformative approach to living. From ancient traditions, notably Buddhism, mindfulness was cultivated to foster clear thinking and serenity. This practice has evolved into a tool for spiritual growth, managing stress, and enhancing overall well-being. By bringing one's attention to experiences occurring in the present moment without judgment, mindfulness can help us mitigate the chaos that life often presents.

The array of techniques under the mindfulness umbrella—including meditation, deep breathing exercises, body scan practices, and mindful movements such as yoga—offers each individual a path that can be personally resonant and profoundly calming. Whether sitting quietly in meditation or moving through yoga poses, these practices help quiet the mind and sharpen our focus on the now.

One of the first steps in adopting mindfulness is understanding why you are drawn to it. For many, the motivation comes from a desire to find relief from anxiety, stress, depression, or simply the overwhelming pace of daily life. Identifying these drivers is critical as they will guide your intentions and help tailor a mindfulness practice that addresses your specific needs.

Setting intentions is not merely about defining what you wish to achieve through mindfulness; it's about committing to a journey of self-discovery and continuous growth. This commitment is essential as it transforms occasional practice into a consistent habit that can significantly impact mental and emotional health.

As we progress through this book, we will delve deeper into how these practices can be seamlessly integrated into your daily routine, how they aid in managing stressors effectively, and how they enhance overall happiness. The ultimate goal is for you to not only learn about these techniques but also experience them so that you feel equipped to face life's challenges with newfound resilience and calm.

This chapter sets the stage for a transformative process by fostering an understanding of mindfulness's roots and its practical applications. It invites you to begin with curiosity and openness, ready to explore how simple acts of awareness can bring about profound changes in your response to everyday stressors. As you move forward, remember that each step taken in mindfulness is a step toward reclaiming your joy and serenity amidst life's inevitable chaos.

At its core, mindfulness is about being fully present in the moment, without judgment or attachment to thoughts or feelings. It involves cultivating awareness of one's thoughts, emotions, and bodily sensations as they arise, allowing for a deeper understanding of oneself and the world around us. By understanding the foundational principles of mindfulness and its historical roots, we can appreciate its significance in promoting overall well-being and mental clarity.

From ancient Eastern philosophies, mindfulness has deep roots in practices like Buddhism and yoga. These traditions emphasize the importance of being present and aware in each moment, recognizing the impermanent nature of life and the interconnectedness of all beings. By learning about the historical origins of mindfulness, we can gain a deeper appreciation for its transformative power in our modern lives.

The essence of mindfulness lies in non-judgmental awareness. This means observing our thoughts and emotions without labeling them as good or bad, right or wrong. Embracing this principle allows us to cultivate inner peace and acceptance, fostering a more compassionate relationship with ourselves and others. Mindfulness also encourages us to let go of attachments to past regrets or future worries, focusing instead on the richness of the present moment.

Understanding that mindfulness is not about achieving a specific state but rather about cultivating a way of being can alleviate any pressure or expectations we may place on ourselves. It is not about clearing the mind of thoughts but rather observing them with curiosity and kindness. By acknowledging that distractions will arise during practice, we can approach mindfulness with a gentle and forgiving attitude toward ourselves.

As we delve into the historical roots and foundational principles of mindfulness, it becomes evident that this practice is not just a passing trend but a profound way of living with intention and awareness. By immersing ourselves in these principles, we open ourselves to a world of personal growth and transformation possibilities. The wisdom passed down through the centuries reminds us that mindfulness is not merely a tool for stress reduction but a profound path toward self-discovery and inner peace.

Exploring the Tapestry of Mindfulness Practices

Mindfulness offers a rich tapestry of techniques to explore, each serving as a pathway to presence and tranquility. Meditation, the cornerstone of mindfulness practices, invites us to observe our thoughts without judgment, cultivating a profound self-awareness. Through meditation, we learn to navigate the landscape of our minds with clarity and compassion. Deep breathing exercises act as anchors, grounding us in the rhythm of each inhale and exhale, providing solace in moments of chaos. We can find stillness amidst the storm by harnessing the power of our breath.

Body scan practices guide us in reconnecting with our physical selves, fostering a profound awareness of sensations and emotions held within our bodies. As we traverse each muscle and joint with mindful attention, we unravel the knots of tension that bind us, inviting relaxation and release. Mindful movements such as yoga offer a harmonious blend of breath and motion, uniting mind, body, and spirit in fluid synchrony. We honor the present moment with grace and gratitude through gentle stretches and intentional poses.

Exploring these diverse techniques allows us to tailor our mindfulness practice to suit our unique preferences and needs. By experimenting with various methods, we can uncover what resonates most deeply within us, forging a personalized path to inner peace. Whether it's the stillness of meditation, the grounding force of deep breathing, the embodied awareness of body scans, or the dynamic flow of mindful movements like yoga, there is a technique waiting to embrace us on our journey toward serenity.

As we delve into the array of mindfulness practices available, we open ourselves to a world of self-discovery and transformation. Each technique offers a gateway to a greater understanding of ourselves and the world around us. Through meditation, we cultivate patience and acceptance; with deep breathing, we find calm amid turmoil; through body scans, we unearth buried emotions awaiting acknowledgment; and through mindful movements, we embody presence and vitality.

Embracing this variety empowers us to navigate life's challenges with resilience and grace. By incorporating mindfulness techniques into our daily routine, we equip ourselves with an arsenal of emotional regulation and stress management tools. The richness of these practices lies in their individual benefits and collective power to nurture a holistic sense of well-being.

In this exploration of mindfulness techniques lies an invitation to embark on a profound inward journey that promises serenity and self-discovery. Each method serves as a stepping stone toward deeper self-awareness and emotional mastery. As we embrace this diversity in practice, we open ourselves up to a world of possibilities where tranquility is not merely a destination but a way of being—a way that beckons us to reclaim joy amidst life's chaos.

As you delve into mindfulness, you must identify your reasons for embarking on this transformative journey. Setting intentions for your practice can provide a clear roadmap toward achieving the peace and serenity you seek daily. Reflecting on why you are drawn to mindfulness can help solidify your commitment and motivation to incorporate these practices into your routine.

Begin by acknowledging your current challenges and struggles. Are you feeling overwhelmed by stress, anxiety, or a constant sense of unease? Recognizing these difficulties is the first step towards seeking a solution through mindfulness. Accepting where you are right now opens the door to exploring new pathways for healing and growth.

Consider the impact of stress on your overall well-being. How does it affect your relationships, work performance, and mental health? Recognizing the toll of stress can be a powerful motivator for embracing mindfulness practices to cope with life's demands more effectively.

Visualize the kind of life you aspire to lead. Envision yourself responding to challenges with calmness, clarity, and resilience. Imagine cultivating a deep inner peace that radiates outwards, positively influencing those around you. This vision can serve as a guiding light as you navigate the complexities of modern living.

Set clear intentions for your mindfulness practice. Whether it's to reduce stress, improve focus, cultivate self-compassion, or enhance emotional regulation, defining your goals can give direction and purpose to your efforts. Clarify what you hope to achieve through mindfulness and outline actionable steps to move closer to those aspirations.

Commit to a regular practice that aligns with your intentions. Consistency is critical, whether starting each day with a brief meditation session, incorporating mindful movement into your routine, or practicing deep breathing exercises during moments of tension. Create a realistic schedule that allows for daily moments of mindfulness, even amidst a busy schedule.

Embrace the journey of self-discovery and growth that mindfulness offers. As you deepen your practice, remain open to new insights about yourself and the world around you. Celebrate small victories, acknowledging your progress in nurturing your inner peace and well-being.

In setting intentions for your mindfulness practice, remember that this is a personal voyage tailored to meet your unique needs and aspirations. Stay compassionate towards yourself, allowing room for setbacks and adjustments as you navigate this path towards greater calmness and clarity in your life.

Awakening to Mindfulness

Through our exploration of mindfulness, we have uncovered its rich historical roots and the diverse techniques that it encompasses. Each method offers unique benefits, from meditation to mindful movement, designed to anchor you in the present and alleviate the whirlwind of daily stress. As you stand at the threshold of this journey, remember that mindfulness is not just a practice but a transformative experience that beckons a deeper understanding of oneself.

Set your intentions with clarity and purpose. Whether you seek tranquility in tumultuous times or a deeper connection with your inner self, mindfulness offers a path tailored just for you. It's about finding what resonates with your personal needs and lifestyle, making your practice as unique as you are.

The steps ahead promise peace, serenity, and an empowered sense of control over your mental and emotional well-being. Embrace these tools—they are simple yet profound ways to enhance your quality of life. Each moment spent in mindfulness is a step toward a more centered and joyful existence.

Encourage yourself to experiment with different mindfulness techniques. Feel the ground under your feet during a walking meditation or notice the subtle changes in your body through a body scan. These practices are designed to be integrated into your daily routine, making mindfulness an accessible ally against the chaos of everyday life.

As we progress in this book, let each page equip you with practical strategies to cultivate calmness and reclaim joy. The journey through mindfulness is as rewarding as the destination, and each step forward is a step toward transforming stress into serenity.

Stay engaged, stay curious, and, most importantly, take these steps at your own pace. Your path to mindfulness is yours to shape—crafted by your intentions, guided by your desires, and enriched by the peace you gather along the way. Let's embark on this transformative journey together, embracing each moment with openness and anticipation for the calm that awaits.

Chapter 2: The Transformative Power of Mindfulness

"The best way to capture moments is to

pay attention. This is how we

cultivate mindfulness."

Jon Kabat-Zinn

Unveiling the Science Behind Mindfulness

Mindfulness is more than just a popular wellness trend; it's a transformative practice backed by extensive scientific research. For anyone feeling overwhelmed by the demands of daily life, understanding how mindfulness can directly benefit mental, emotional, and physical health is crucial. This exploration reveals that mindfulness isn't merely about quieting the mind; it's about harnessing a tool that can fundamentally enhance the quality of life.

Scientific studies confirm that mindfulness meditation reduces stress and anxiety by altering the brain's response to stress triggers. It down-regulates the neurological pathways associated with stress reactions and up-regulates those involved with calmness and emotional regulation. This shift not only helps in managing immediate stressors but also contributes to long-term emotional resilience. This can be a game-changer for anyone struggling to keep their head above water in a sea of responsibilities.

Moreover, mindfulness enhances focus and concentration. In our digital age, where distractions are a constant, the ability to focus is more valuable than ever. Mindfulness training has improved the brain's ability to ignore distractions, leading to greater productivity and efficiency at work and home. This isn't just about getting more done; it's about enhancing the quality of what we do and feeling less scattered in our efforts.

Emotional regulation is another significant benefit of regular mindfulness practice. By fostering an increased awareness of one's thoughts and feelings, mindfulness allows individuals to recognize patterns that may lead to reactive behaviors. This awareness creates a space between stimulus and response where the choice lies—enabling more measured, thoughtful interactions that lead to healthier personal and professional relationships.

Transforming Relationships Through Awareness

The impact of mindfulness extends beyond self-improvement—it also improves how we relate to others. By reducing reactivity, mindfulness encourages responses based on conscious choices rather than impulsive emotions. This can significantly enhance relationships with family members, friends, or colleagues, leading to more harmonious interactions and a supportive social environment.

Understanding these benefits positions you to make informed decisions about incorporating mindfulness into your life. It's not just about finding time to meditate; it's about integrating mindful moments throughout your day—whether taking three deep breaths before responding in a meeting or noticing the sensations of your feet on the ground as you walk.

Practical Steps Toward a Mindful Life

To begin integrating mindfulness into your routine, start small. Dedicate five minutes each morning or evening to sit quietly and focus on your breath. When your mind wanders—and it will—gently guide it back without judgment. This simple practice can be the foundation for deeper exploring mindfulness techniques and their benefits.

Remember, the journey toward mindfulness is personal and

unique for everyone. What works for one person might not work for another; thus, exploring various methods is crucial in discovering what helps you connect with a sense of calm and centeredness.

By embracing mindfulness, you're not just coping with chaos—you're transforming how you experience it. You're equipping yourself with tools to survive and thrive amidst life's challenges. Engage actively with these strategies; they hold the potential for personal transformation and reshaping your interactions with the world around you.

Mindfulness is not merely a trendy concept but a scientifically proven method to enhance mental, emotional, and physical well-being. Research has shown that regular mindfulness practice can lead to many benefits that positively impact various aspects of our lives. The effects of mindfulness are profound and far-reaching, from reducing stress and anxiety to improving focus, concentration, and emotional regulation.

One of the key benefits of mindfulness is its ability to reduce stress and anxiety levels. Individuals can effectively manage their response to stressors by cultivating present-moment awareness, leading to a calmer and more centered state of mind. Studies have demonstrated that mindfulness practices can lower cortisol levels, the hormone associated with stress, promoting relaxation and overall well-being.

Moreover, mindfulness enhances focus and concentration by training the mind to stay present and attentive. Regular practice can sharpen cognitive abilities, improve memory retention, and increase mental clarity. By immersing ourselves in the present moment without judgment, we can heighten our awareness and optimize our cognitive functions for better productivity and performance.

Emotional regulation is another significant benefit of mindfulness practice. By developing a non-reactive stance towards our emotions, we can learn to observe them without becoming overwhelmed or consumed. This skill enables us to respond thoughtfully rather than impulsively in challenging situations, fostering healthier relationships and improved communication.

Additionally, mindfulness fosters resilience by nurturing an inner strength that allows individuals to bounce back from setbacks more quickly. Through mindful awareness, we can build emotional resilience by acknowledging our experiences without getting entangled in negative thought patterns or self-criticism. This resilience equips us to navigate life's ups and downs with grace and adaptability.

Cultivating Focus, Emotional Regulation, and Resilience through Mindfulness

Mindfulness practice offers a powerful tool for enhancing focus, emotional regulation, and resilience in our daily lives. By cultivating mindfulness, we can sharpen our attention and concentration, allowing us to engage more fully in the present moment. Mindfulness lets us eliminate distractions and hone in on the task, increasing productivity and efficiency. We can train our minds to be more alert and attentive through regular practice, fostering a deep sense of clarity and mental acuity.

Emotional regulation is another significant benefit of mindfulness practice. By developing awareness of our thoughts and feelings without judgment, we can better understand and manage our emotions. Mindfulness teaches us to observe our internal experiences with a sense of curiosity and compassion rather than reacting impulsively. This heightened self-awareness empowers us to respond to challenging situations with more remarkable composure and calmness, fostering emotional resilience in adversity.

Resilience, the ability to bounce back from setbacks and adapt to life's challenges, is a crucial outcome of regular mindfulness practice. We can navigate difficult circumstances gracefully and with grit by cultivating a present-moment awareness and acceptance of change. Mindfulness equips us with the tools to approach obstacles calmly and steadily, enabling us to persevere amid uncertainty and upheaval.

Practical strategies such as mindful breathing exercises, body scans, or loving-kindness meditations can help bolster our focus, emotional regulation, and resilience. These simple yet effective techniques can be integrated seamlessly into our daily routines, providing us with moments of reprieve and reflection amidst the chaos of modern life. By incorporating mindfulness practices into our day-to-day activities, we can gradually rewire our brains for greater attentional control, emotional balance, and adaptive coping mechanisms.

Consistency is critical when it comes to reaping the benefits of mindfulness. Regular practice strengthens neural pathways associated with focus, emotional regulation, and resilience, leading to lasting positive mental and emotional well-being changes. As we commit to nurturing these qualities through mindfulness, we pave the way for a more centered, resilient, and emotionally intelligent way of being in the world.

Mindfulness is a potent catalyst for enhancing our cognitive abilities, emotional well-being, and adaptive capacities. Through dedicated practice, we can harness the transformative power of mindfulness to cultivate a profound sense of presence, stability, and inner strength. By embracing mindfulness as a way of life rather than a mere technique or tool, we open ourselves to a world of growth, healing, and self-discovery possibilities.

Mindfulness Framework: Pathway to Well-being

To understand the transformative power of mindfulness on relationships and overall well-being, let's delve into a conceptual model that illustrates the journey from mindfulness practice to health outcomes. At the base of this model lie mindfulness techniques such as meditation and mindful breathing. These practices are the foundation for the entire process, initiating a cascade of positive mental, emotional, and physical health effects.

Moving up the model, we encounter the intricate neural pathways mindfulness practices affect. Through mechanisms like neuroplasticity and stress reduction, these techniques reshape the brain's structure and function. Studies have shown how consistent mindfulness can lead to tangible changes in brain activity, promoting cognitive flexibility and emotional regulation.

As we progress further, we reach the realm of intermediate outcomes. Here, improved focus, enhanced emotional regulation and heightened resilience become apparent. Mindfulness equips individuals with the tools to navigate daily challenges with clarity and composure, fostering a sense of empowerment in managing life's ups and downs.

The pinnacle of this model showcases the long-term benefits reaped from sustained mindfulness practice. Reduced anxiety levels, enhanced relationship quality, and an overall sense of well-being emerge as natural consequences of embracing mindfulness. Research supports these claims, highlighting how mindfulness cultivates a greater capacity for compassion, empathy, and connection with others.

This framework not only elucidates the progression from practice to outcomes but also serves as a roadmap for readers seeking to integrate mindfulness into their lives effectively. By understanding the intricate connections between each stage of the model, individuals can grasp how incremental changes in their daily routines can lead to profound improvements in their mental and emotional well-being over time.

This conceptual model underscores mindfulness's profound impact on relationships and overall well-being. By incorporating mindfulness practices into daily life and embracing its transformative potential, individuals can cultivate resilience, emotional intelligence, and a profound sense of inner peace that radiates outward into their interactions.

The evidence is compelling: mindfulness holds transformative power for enhancing our lives on multiple levels. By embracing this practice, you can significantly reduce stress and anxiety, which are all too familiar in our fast-paced world. More than just a tool for managing stress, mindfulness enhances your ability to focus and regulate emotions, fostering a resilience that helps you navigate life's challenges gracefully.

Mindfulness isn't just about personal benefits; it also positively affects how we interact with others. Increasing your self-awareness and emotional understanding paves the way for healthier, more compassionate relationships. This improves your connections and contributes to a more empathetic society.

You are capable of mastering these practices. Start small, integrating mindfulness exercises into your daily routine. Whether it's a few minutes of breathing exercises in the morning or a brief meditation session during your lunch break, each step is a move towards greater well-being.

Remember, the journey to mindfulness is not about perfection but progress. Each moment of mindfulness adds up, creating profound changes over time. As you continue to practice, you'll likely notice subtle yet powerful shifts in your mental clarity and emotional stability—ripple effects that enhance every area of your life.

Let this be your invitation to start a practice that could redefine the quality of your life. Engage actively with mindfulness techniques; they are simple yet powerful tools that promise significant rewards. Your path to a calmer, more centered life is within reach—embrace it with open arms and an open heart.

Chapter 3: Breathing Your Way to Serenity

"Feelings come and go like clouds in a windy sky.

Conscious breathing is my anchor."

Thich Nhat Hanh

Unravel the Power of Breath: A Gateway to Inner Peace

Amid our bustling lives, where chaos often reigns supreme, finding a moment of serenity can seem like a distant dream. Yet, the journey to achieving tranquility and a centered mind might be just a breath away. Mindfulness meditation is not just a practice but a profound experience that reconnects us with the essence of our being through the simple act of breathing. This chapter delves deep into how you can harness this powerful tool to face the turbulence of daily life and thrive within it.

At its core, mindfulness meditation invites you to pause and engage in the present moment with kindness and without judgment. It's about noticing where, what you're doing, and how you feel without trying to change anything. For many, this practice begins with something we do every moment of our lives yet rarely pay attention to—our breath. Focusing on breathing helps settle the mind and serves as an anchor to the present, providing a break from the relentless pace of thoughts about the past or worries about the future.

The first lesson here is straightforward: mastering the basics of mindfulness meditation with an emphasis on breath. This involves learning to observe your breathing pattern and recognize its rhythm, depth, and sensations in your body. Such awareness cultivates a peaceful mind, allowing stress and anxiety to dissipate naturally.

Moving beyond the cushion or meditation mat, mindfulness doesn't have to end when your session ends. The second critical insight is about incorporating mindfulness into your daily routines, both formally and informally. This means finding moments throughout your day—during a coffee break while commuting or waiting in line—to center yourself through mindful breathing. These practices reinforce your ability to remain calm and collected amidst daily pressures.

However, beginning meditators often face hurdles that might make them question their progress or even deter them from continuing. The third critical learning point addresses these common challenges, such as dealing with distractions, managing boredom, or handling frustration when meditation doesn't go as planned. Understanding these as part of the journey helps in developing resilience and patience.

Step into Serenity: A Practical Guide to Mindful Breathing

Step 1: Find a Quiet Space

Ensure your meditation area is free from interruptions. A peaceful corner where you feel at ease significantly enhances your ability to focus and relax.

Step 2: Get into a Comfortable Position

Whether seated or lying down, comfort is critical. Keep your back straight yet relaxed. Allow your body to feel supported by the ground or seat beneath you.

Step 3: Bring Your Attention to Your Breath

Initiate with deep breaths, and then let them flow naturally. Concentrate on each inhalation and exhalation, noting how your body moves with each breath.

Step 4: Notice Your Thoughts and Sensations

Acknowledge any thoughts or feelings that arise without engaging with them. Let them pass as you would watch cars on a highway, always returning your focus gently back to your breath.

Step 5: Practice Non-Judgment and Patience

Be kind to yourself if concentration wavers—it's part of learning. Meditation is not about perfection but presence.

Step 6: End Your Meditation Practice

Keep out of your practice by gently moving your extremities before opening your eyes. Carry forward gratitude for this moment of peace as you transition back into daily activities.

Through these steps and insights shared in this chapter, readers are equipped with knowledge and practical tools to find calm amid chaos. By repeatedly returning to these practices, each cultivates their sanctuary within—turning what seems chaotic into an opportunity for growth and serenity.

Mindfulness meditation is a powerful tool that can help you find calm amidst the chaos of daily life. Focusing on your breath can anchor you in the present moment and cultivate inner peace. Attention to your breath can help quiet the mind and reduce stress and anxiety. When you feel overwhelmed or scattered, taking a few moments to focus on your breath can bring you back to the center.

To master the basics of mindfulness meditation focusing on the breath, find a quiet space where you won't be disturbed. Sit comfortably on a cushion on the floor or in a chair with your feet flat on the ground. Close your eyes and begin to pay attention to your breath. Notice the sensation of air entering and leaving your nostrils or the rise and fall of your chest and abdomen.

As you focus on your breath, thoughts will inevitably arise. This is normal and part of the practice. When you notice your mind wandering, gently bring your attention back to your breath. You don't need to judge yourself for getting distracted; acknowledge the thought and return to focusing on your breath.

Start with short sessions of 5-10 minutes. As you become more comfortable with the practice, you can gradually increase the length of your sessions. Consistency is vital, so try to meditate at the same time each day to establish a routine. Over time, you may notice a greater sense of calm and clarity in your daily life as you incorporate this practice into your routine.

Embracing Mindfulness: A Transformative Journey

Incorporating mindfulness meditation into your daily routines, formally and informally, can be a transformative practice that helps you cultivate inner peace amidst life's chaos. Integrating mindfulness into daily activities can enhance well-being and manage stress more effectively. Here are some practical strategies to help you seamlessly weave mindfulness into your daily life:

Start Your Day Mindfully

Begin each morning with a few minutes of mindful breathing to set a positive tone for the day ahead. Take deep breaths, focusing on the sensation of air entering and leaving your body. This simple practice can center your mind and prepare you to face any challenges with clarity and calmness.

Infuse Mindfulness into Routine Tasks

Turn routine activities like washing dishes, walking, or eating into opportunities for mindfulness. Engage all your senses in the present moment. Notice the warmth of water on your hands, the sound of birds chirping, or the taste of each bite of food. By immersing yourself fully in these experiences, you can cultivate peace and gratitude in everyday moments.

Schedule Formal Meditation Sessions

Set aside dedicated time each day for formal meditation practice. Find a quiet space where you won't be disturbed and focus on your breath or body sensations. Start with a few minutes and gradually increase the duration as you build consistency. Regular formal meditation sessions can deepen your mindfulness practice and promote emotional resilience.

Practice Mindful Listening

During conversations with others, practice active listening by giving them your full attention without judgment or distraction. Focus on their words, tone, and body language. This mindful listening can foster deeper connections with others and enhance your communication skills.

Take Mindful Breaks

Throughout the day, pause for mindful breaks to check in with yourself and recenter your thoughts. Close your eyes for a moment, take a few deep breaths, and notice how you feel physically and emotionally. These brief moments of mindfulness can help you stay grounded amidst busyness and stress.

Cultivate Gratitude through Mindfulness

Integrate gratitude practices into your daily routine by reflecting on moments of joy or blessings. Take time each day to acknowledge what you're grateful for a supportive friend, a beautiful sunset, or a small personal achievement. This mindful gratitude can shift your perspective towards positivity and abundance.

End Your Day Mindfully

Close each day with a brief mindfulness practice to unwind and prepare for restful sleep. Reflect on the day's events without judgment, acknowledging challenges and moments of joy. Engaging in this reflective practice can promote relaxation and mental clarity before bedtime.

By incorporating mindfulness meditation into formal sessions and everyday activities, you can nurture a sense of calmness and presence throughout your day. Embrace these practical strategies to infuse mindfulness into your routines effortlessly, fostering emotional well-being and resilience in the face of life's demands.

As you venture into mindfulness meditation, it's common to encounter challenges that can hinder your progress and discourage you from continuing. However, these obstacles are natural parts of the learning process and can be overcome with patience and perseverance. One common challenge faced by beginners during meditation is the wandering mind. Thoughts drift in and out, disrupting your focus on the present moment, and remembering that this is normal and not a sign of failure is essential.

To overcome this challenge, gently guide your attention to your breath whenever you notice your mind wandering.

Acknowledge the thoughts without judgment and then return your focus to the sensation of breathing. Gradually, with practice, you'll find it easier to maintain concentration and experience moments of stillness and calmness.

Another obstacle many beginners face is restlessness or discomfort in the body. Sitting still for an extended period can lead to physical pain, which can be distracting during meditation. To address this, ensure you are sitting comfortably with good posture, allowing your body to relax while remaining alert. You can also try incorporating gentle movements or stretching before your meditation session to release any tension.

Furthermore, impatience is a common challenge when individuals expect immediate results from their meditation practice. It's important to understand that mindfulness is a skill that develops over time. Patience is critical in allowing yourself the space to grow and evolve in your practice. Rather than focusing on achieving specific outcomes, embrace the process of learning and self-discovery that comes with each session.

Additionally, frustration or self-criticism may arise when you perceive your meditation practice as not meeting expectations. Remember that there is no right or wrong way to meditate; each session is an opportunity for growth and learning. Be compassionate towards yourself, acknowledging that progress takes time and effort. Celebrate small victories along the way, no matter how insignificant.

Moreover, finding time for regular meditation sessions amidst a busy schedule can be challenging for beginners. Incorporating mindfulness into daily routines can help make it more manageable. Short moments of mindfulness during everyday activities, such as focusing on the sensations of washing dishes or walking mindfully, can be just as beneficial as longer formal sessions.

Lastly, maintaining consistency in your practice can be difficult when faced with competing priorities or wavering motivation. Establishing a routine by setting aside dedicated time each day for meditation can help create a sense of discipline and commitment. Start with small achievable goals, gradually increasing the duration or frequency of your sessions as you become more comfortable with the practice.

By acknowledging these common challenges and implementing practical strategies to overcome them, you can cultivate a more resilient and fulfilling meditation practice. Remember that progress is not linear, and each moment of presence contributes to your growth toward inner peace and serenity.

Mindfulness meditation is more than just a practice; it's a transformative journey towards serenity that you can embark on every day, even amidst the chaos of life. By mastering the basics of focusing on your breath, you've taken the first essential step to calm your mind and anchor yourself in the present moment.

Harness the Power of Routine

Incorporating mindfulness into your daily routines doesn't have to be a daunting task. Whether it's a few minutes of deep breathing before starting your day or a quick mindfulness pause before responding to stressful situations, each small step is a building block toward greater emotional resilience and mental clarity. Remember, consistency is vital. The more regularly you practice, the more natural it will become, seamlessly blending into the fabric of your daily life.

Overcome Challenges with Confidence

It's common to face hurdles at the beginning of your meditation journey. Distractions, restlessness, or self-doubt might surface, but these are not setbacks—they are part of the learning curve. Each challenge is an opportunity to grow and strengthen your practice. When difficulties arise, gently remind yourself that meditation is a skill that improves with practice and patience.

Take Action

Now is the perfect time to take control of your well-being through mindfulness meditation. With each breath you take, you can bring more peace and joy into your life. Start small, stay consistent, and be patient with yourself as you discover the calming effects of this profound practice.

Your Path Forward

As you continue on this path, remember that every moment offers a new chance to engage mindfully. Let this practice be your steady companion as you navigate life's complexities. Trust in your ability to cultivate serenity within yourself—it is one of the most empowering gifts you can offer yourself and those around you.

Embrace this journey with openness, knowing that each mindful breath is a step towards reclaiming joy and tranquility in your life.

Chapter 4: Crafting Your Mindfulness Routine

"Mindfulness means being awake. It means

knowing what you are doing."

Jon Kabat-Zinn

Unleash the Power of Now: A Practical Blueprint

Amidst the relentless pace of modern life, finding moments of calm can seem like a quest for a mirage. However, mindfulness offers a beacon of tranquility in the tumult of daily chaos. By weaving mindfulness into the fabric of everyday activities, you can transform mundane routines into opportunities for serenity and self-discovery. This transformative journey begins with the understanding that mindfulness is not merely a practice, but a way of being that can infuse every action with intention and awareness.

Mindfulness is an accessible tool designed to bring balance and focus to your life. It involves being present in each moment, observing thoughts and sensations without attachment or judgment. The beauty of mindfulness lies in its simplicity and universality—anyone can practice it anywhere without needing special equipment or extensive training. The key is to start small, integrating mindful awareness into routine activities like eating, walking, or commuting. These are moments often lost to auto-pilot; by reclaiming them, you cultivate a heightened sense of living that gradually permeates all aspects of your life.

For those constantly juggling demands and deadlines, developing a personalized mindfulness routine that fits into a busy schedule may seem daunting. Yet, mindfulness can bring the most significant relief and clarity in these packed schedules. The first step is identifying daily activities where mindfulness can be seamlessly integrated. This could be as simple as turning your morning shower into a sensory experience where you fully engage with the feel of water on your skin or droplets hitting the floor.

Next is setting an intentional mindset before beginning any activity. Remind yourself to stay present and fully engage with whatever you are doing. It's about shifting from being 'mind full' to being mindful. This intention acts like an anchor, helping you stay focused amidst distractions and reconnecting with the task at hand whenever you drift away.

The core practice involves cultivating awareness and presence during these activities. Notice when your mind wanders and gently guide it to the present moment. This isn't about suppression or harsh self-judgment but about observing with curiosity and openness.

Mindful breathing is another potent tool in this arsenal. Using breath as an anchor keeps you rooted in the now, which is especially useful when emotions or stress levels spike. Deep breaths can recalibrate your mental state, allowing you to approach situations with fresh eyes.

Extending Mindfulness Beyond Meditation

As your comfort with these practices grows, extend mindfulness to other parts of your day. Each step becomes an opportunity to deepen self-awareness and enhance quality of life. Reflect on these experiences regularly; recognize how they affect your mood, stress levels, and overall well-being.

Finally, consider this process not as adding another task to your day but as transforming existing ones into moments of connection with yourself. This shift in perspective reduces feelings of busyness and overload because each action becomes more purposeful and centered.

Mindful Moments: Everyday Practice for Peaceful Living

Identify Daily Activities for Mindfulness Integration

- Reflect on routines ideal for incorporating mindfulness.
- Opt for repetitive tasks where focus can be easily maintained.

Set an Intention for Mindfulness

- Begin each activity with a clear intent to remain present.
- Engage all senses and release distractions as they arise.

Cultivate Awareness and Presence

- Keep attention anchored in the current activity.
- Return focus gently when it drifts away.

Practice Mindful Breathing

- Use breaths as focal points during tasks.
- Re-center through breathing when overwhelmed.

Extend Mindfulness to Other Activities

- Gradually include more daily actions under this mindful approach.
- Maintain curiosity and non-judgment throughout practices.

Reflect on the Benefits of Mindful Integration

- Evaluate how mindfulness impacts mental clarity and emotional stability.
- Acknowledge growth areas and refine practices accordingly.

By embedding these steps into your daily life, you pave the way toward sustained peace and heightened awareness—turning every moment into an opportunity for growth and tranquility.

Incorporating mindfulness practices into your daily routine doesn't have to be complicated or time-consuming. You can seamlessly integrate mindfulness into your everyday activities, transforming mundane moments into opportunities for peace and presence. Start by bringing your awareness to the present moment during routine tasks like brushing your teeth, showering, or preparing a meal. Notice the sensations, sounds, and movements involved in these activities without judgment or distraction.

Practice mindful breathing throughout the day to anchor

yourself in the present moment. Take a few deep breaths, focusing on the sensation of air entering and leaving your body. This simple practice can help calm your mind and center your thoughts, even amid a hectic day. Mindful breathing can be done anytime, anywhere, making it a versatile tool for cultivating mindfulness in various situations.

Engage all your senses during daily activities to enhance mindfulness. Whether eating a meal, walking in nature, or sitting at your desk, pay attention to the sights, sounds, smells, tastes, and textures around you. By immersing yourself fully in the sensory experience of each moment, you can deepen your connection to the present and cultivate a sense of gratitude for the richness of life.

Create mindful transitions between different tasks or activities to maintain a sense of continuity and presence throughout your day. Before moving on to a new task, take a moment to pause, breathe deeply, and reset your focus. This practice can help prevent feelings of overwhelm or scattered attention by grounding you in the present moment before proceeding with the next activity.

Use reminders or cues to prompt mindfulness throughout your day. Set alarms on your phone, place sticky notes strategically, or link mindfulness practices to specific triggers like entering a room or answering a phone call. These gentle reminders can help you stay attuned to the present moment and reinforce your commitment to cultivating mindfulness daily.

Crafting Your Personalized Mindfulness Routine

Finding time for mindfulness practices can seem like an additional burden amid a bustling schedule. However, creating a personalized mindfulness routine that fits seamlessly into your daily life is achievable and essential for maintaining a sense of calm and balance. You can reap the benefits of increased clarity, emotional stability, and overall well-being by tailoring your mindfulness practice to suit your unique needs and schedule.

Start by setting aside dedicated time each day for your mindfulness practice. This could be as little as five minutes in the morning or before bed. Consistency is vital, so choose a time that works best for you and commit to it daily. Incorporating mindfulness into your routines, such as during your commute, while waiting in line, or even during short breaks at work, can help make it a natural part of your day.

Experiment with different mindfulness techniques to find what resonates most with you. Whether it's mindful breathing exercises, body scans, guided meditations, or mindful movements like yoga or tai chi, exploring various practices can help you discover what suits you best. Remember that there is no one-size-fits-all approach to mindfulness, so feel free to mix and match techniques until you find what feels most comfortable and practical for you.

Keep your mindfulness practice simple and accessible. You

don't need fancy equipment or a specific setting to practice mindfulness effectively. Find a quiet space where you feel comfortable, whether it's a corner of your home, a park bench, or even a quiet room at work. Engage your senses by noticing the sights, sounds, smells, and sensations around you. Allow yourself to be fully present in the moment without judgment or attachment to thoughts or feelings that arise.

Integrate mindfulness into everyday activities to make it a seamless routine. Practice mindful eating by savoring each bite and noticing your food's flavors and textures. Bring awareness to daily tasks like washing dishes or showering, focusing on the sensations and movements involved. Mindful walking can also be a powerful practice, allowing you to connect with nature and ground yourself in the present moment.

Reflect on the impact of your mindfulness practice regularly. Notice any changes in your mood, stress levels, relationships, or overall outlook. Journaling can be a helpful tool for tracking your progress and gaining insights into how mindfulness positively influences various areas of your life. Celebrate small victories along the way, acknowledging the effort you put into nurturing your well-being through mindfulness.

Remember that self-compassion is critical in developing a sustainable mindfulness routine. Be gentle with yourself if you miss a day or struggle with consistency. Instead of viewing it as a failure, see it as an opportunity to learn and grow in your practice. Approach each day with curiosity and openness, embracing whatever arises with kindness and acceptance.

Incorporating mindfulness into your busy schedule may initially seem challenging, but with dedication and flexibility, you can create a routine that nourishes your mind, body, and spirit. Embrace the journey of self-discovery and transformation through mindfulness practice, knowing that each moment of presence brings you closer to inner peace and resilience in the face of life's challenges.

Incorporating mindfulness exercises into your daily routine can significantly enhance your moment-to-moment awareness, leading to a more present and grounded life experience. One powerful exercise to cultivate mindfulness is the body scan. This practice involves systematically bringing attention to each body part, starting from the toes and moving up to the crown of your head. You can connect deeply with your body and the present moment by tuning into physical sensations without judgment.

Another effective mindfulness exercise is mindful breathing. Simply focusing on the rhythm of your breath can anchor you in the present and calm a busy mind. As you inhale and exhale, notice the sensations of each breath without trying to change them. This practice can help regulate emotions, reduce stress, and increase overall well-being by fostering a sense of inner peace.

Mindful walking is a powerful way to engage with your surroundings and reconnect with the present moment. Pay attention to each step, feeling the ground beneath your feet and observing the sights and sounds around you. Walking mindfully can be especially beneficial when feeling overwhelmed or stressed, providing a grounding anchor in times of turbulence.

Practicing gratitude is another mindfulness exercise that can shift your focus from what's lacking in life to what you already have. Take a few moments each day to reflect on three things you are grateful for, big or small. This practice can cultivate a positive outlook, enhance resilience, and foster a more profound sense of contentment in daily life.

Engaging in mindful listening is essential for building deeper connections with others and fostering empathy. When in conversation, practice genuinely listening to the speaker without interrupting or formulating responses in your mind. You strengthen relationships and sharpen your presence and awareness by giving your full attention to the speaker's words and nonverbal cues.

Mindful eating is a transformative practice that involves savoring each bite of food with full attention. By slowing down during meals, engaging all your senses, and appreciating the flavors and textures of your food, you can cultivate a healthier relationship with eating and deepen your connection to nourishment.

Incorporating these mindfulness exercises into your daily routine can lead to profound shifts in how you experience life. Dedicating even just a few minutes each day to these practices can enhance your moment-to-moment awareness, reduce stress levels, improve emotional regulation, and cultivate a greater sense of peace and well-being. Remember that mindfulness is not about perfection but progress; every moment you engage with these exercises brings you closer to living with intention and presence.

Mindfulness is more than just a practice; it's a transformative approach that seamlessly integrates into every moment of your daily life. By now, you have explored various ways to weave mindfulness into your routine activities, ensuring you can maintain a sense of calm and presence even amidst a hectic schedule. The key is not to see mindfulness as an additional task on your to-do list but as a subtle shift in how you engage with everyday tasks.

You can develop a personalized mindfulness routine that respects the realities of your busy life. Remember, the goal is not perfection but progress. Small, consistent steps are what lead to lasting changes. Whether taking a few deep breaths before starting your car or feeling the texture of the soap as you wash dishes, these moments accumulate to enhance your overall well-being.

Moreover, mindfulness exercises to boost moment-to-moment awareness can dramatically improve focus and reduce stress. These practices don't require secluded meditation for hours; they are about finding peace throughout your day. It's about being present rather than doing perfectly.

As you move forward, take these strategies and adapt them as needed. Your journey towards mindfulness isn't static; it evolves with your life's rhythms and needs. Trust in your ability to cultivate serenity within yourself—a powerful tool supporting you in all aspects of life.

Finally, remember that every step in this journey enhances your peace and sets a profound example for those around you. By embodying mindfulness, you encourage others to explore their paths to tranquility and joy. So keep moving forward with kindness and patience for yourself, celebrating each moment of awareness as a victory in its own right.

Chapter 5: Mindfulness in Motion

"In today's rush, we all think too much, seek too

much, want too much and forget about

the joy of just being."

Eckhart Tolle

Unleash the Power of Your Body to Quiet Your Mind

Understanding the profound connection between physical movement and mental well-being is essential for anyone seeking tranquility in today's fast-paced world. Mindfulness in motion—engaging in physical activities with a mindful awareness—offers a dynamic way to anchor yourself in the present moment while rejuvenating your mind and body. This approach can be particularly transformative for individuals who find traditional seated meditation challenging or wish to add variety to their mindfulness practices.

The essence of mindfulness exercises lies in their ability to draw our attention away from the chaotic swirl of thoughts and worries, focusing instead on the here and now. Incorporating movements such as yoga, tai chi, or even mindful walking into your routine creates opportunities for your body to assist your mind in pursuing peace. These activities are not just physical exercises; they are forms of moving meditation that enhance your awareness of bodily sensations, breathing patterns, and the surrounding environment.

One of the first steps to integrating these practices is to discover which form of mindful movement resonates most with you. Whether it's the gentle flow of yoga poses, the disciplined movements of tai chi, or the simple rhythm of walking, each activity offers unique benefits and pathways to presence. It's essential to approach these practices with curiosity and without judgment, allowing yourself the space to explore how each movement feels in your body.

As you begin incorporating these exercises into your daily life, consider setting aside specific times to engage in uninterrupted activities. Even a few minutes can make a significant difference. Over time, this dedicated practice can help you develop a deeper connection to your physical self while fostering mental clarity and emotional resilience.

You understand why these activities aid mindfulness and can enhance motivation and commitment. Physical movement has been shown to reduce stress hormones like cortisol and increase endorphins, improving mood and alleviating anxiety. Engaging in mindful movements also encourages you to break away from automatic pilot mode, enriching your everyday actions with an enriching layer of intentionality.

It is also beneficial to create a personal space that encourages mindfulness practice. This might be a specific room or a corner with a yoga mat and calming elements such as candles or soothing artwork. The environment you create can significantly influence your ability to connect deeply with your practice.

Finally, remember that mindfulness in motion is about finding joy and serenity through action. It's not about performance or achieving perfection but about embracing each moment with acceptance and awareness. As you move and breathe consciously, you'll likely find that your mind is more straightforward and you have more energy and enthusiasm for other aspects of life.

Through engaging directly with these strategies—discovering enjoyable mindful movements, integrating them regularly into your routine, understanding their benefits on a deeper level, and creating supportive environments—you empower yourself to transform stress into serenity actively. Each step forward in this journey brings you closer to reclaiming joy in your life by establishing a harmonious balance between body and mind.

Mindfulness exercises are like a mirror reflecting the present moment, allowing us to observe our thoughts and emotions without judgment. They serve as anchors, grounding us in the now amidst life's chaos. One powerful way to deepen our mindfulness is through mindful movements and exercises. These practices invite us to cultivate awareness through physical movement, connecting our bodies and minds in the present moment.

Discovering mindful movements can be a transformative experience. Activities like yoga, tai chi, or walking meditation offer opportunities to synchronize breath with movement, fostering a sense of unity within ourselves. Engaging in these practices promotes flexibility, strength, and balance not only in the body but also in the mind. As we move intentionally and with awareness, we learn to appreciate the beauty of each moment as it unfolds.

Exploring these exercises can unveil a new dimension of mindfulness that transcends sitting meditation and extends into our daily actions. Incorporating mindful movements into our routine infuses our lives with presence and intentionality. These exercises become reminders to slow down, breathe deeply, and fully immerse ourselves in whatever task.

Mindful movements offer a gateway to present-moment awareness. They encourage us to let go of distractions and focus on the sensations arising within our bodies. Through deliberate movement and conscious breathing, we learn to quiet the mind's chatter and attune ourselves to the richness of each moment. This heightened awareness can lead to profound insights and a deeper connection with ourselves.

As you explore mindful movements, notice how they enhance

your mindfulness practice. Pay attention to how your body feels during these activities, how your breath guides your movements, and how your mind responds to the experience. Allow yourself to be fully present in each posture or step, embracing the sensations that arise without attachment or aversion.

Elevating Mindfulness Through Movement

Integrating activities like yoga, tai chi, or walking meditation into your mindfulness practice can significantly enhance your ability to stay present and grounded amid daily chaos. These movement-based practices offer a dynamic way to connect your mind and body, fostering a more profound sense of awareness and relaxation.

Yoga, with its focus on breathwork and gentle movements, can help you tune into the sensations of your body and quiet the chatter of the mind. By flowing through poses that require concentration and balance, you learn to be fully present in each moment, letting go of worries about the past or future.

Tai chi, often described as "meditation in motion," combines slow, deliberate movements with deep breathing to cultivate mindfulness. The fluid motions of tai chi encourage a state of calm alertness, allowing you to release tension and stress while improving physical balance and coordination.

Walking meditation is a simple yet powerful practice that

involves bringing your full attention to each step you take. Walking mindfully indoors and outdoors can help you slow down, appreciate your environment, and center yourself in the present moment.

By incorporating these mindful movement practices into your daily routine, you create opportunities to step away from the demands of life and reconnect with yourself on a deeper level. Each session becomes a sanctuary where you can let go of distractions and immerse yourself in the experience of moving with intention and awareness.

Physical movement is not just about keeping the body healthy; it plays a crucial role in maintaining mental well-being. The connection between physical activity and mental health is profound, with movement serving as a powerful tool for managing stress, anxiety, and low moods. When we engage in activities that get our bodies moving, whether through yoga, tai chi, walking meditation, or any form of exercise, we release endorphins - the body's natural mood enhancers. These feel-good chemicals can help alleviate feelings of tension and promote a sense of well-being.

Regular physical activity has been shown to reduce symptoms of anxiety and depression, making it an essential component of a holistic approach to mental wellness. By incorporating mindful movement practices into your routine, you can tap into the inherent connection between physical and psychological health. Exercise boosts your mood and improves cognitive function, enhancing your ability to focus and concentrate. This dual benefit of physical activity underscores its significance in promoting overall well-being.

Engaging in mindful movement can also help cultivate present-moment awareness, similar to other mindfulness practices like meditation or deep breathing exercises. By focusing on the sensations in your body as you move, you anchor yourself in the present moment, allowing distractions to fade away. This heightened awareness can lead to greater clarity and calmness, helping you navigate daily challenges with more resilience and composure.

The mind-body connection is a powerful force, and when we nurture both aspects through physical movement, we create a harmonious balance that supports our overall health. Movement can be a form of self-expression, allowing us to release pent-up emotions or stress affecting our mental state. Whether through gentle stretches or more vigorous workouts, finding ways to move your body mindfully can be transformative for your emotional well-being.

It's essential to listen to your body during physical activity and honor its needs. Pushing yourself too hard can lead to burnout or injury, which may adversely affect your mental health. Finding a balance between challenging yourself and practicing self-care is critical to reaping the full benefits of mindful movement. Remember that every step you take towards caring for your body is also a step towards nurturing your mind.

Incorporating physical movement into your mindfulness practice can enhance effectiveness, offering a dynamic approach to cultivating inner peace and presence. Whether you practice yoga poses that focus on breath awareness or engage in flowing tai chi movements that encourage relaxation, each moment spent moving with intention brings you closer to balance and tranquility. By embracing the synergy between physical activity and mental well-being, you open yourself to a world of possibilities where resilience, joy, and peace are within reach by simply moving your body with mindfulness.

As we've explored the profound interconnection between physical movement and mental well-being, it's clear that incorporating mindful exercises like yoga, tai chi, or walking meditation can significantly enhance your mindfulness practice. These activities not only ground you in the present moment but also offer numerous health benefits beyond mental tranquility.

Mindful movements are a practical tool for staying centered amidst the daily chaos. By engaging in these exercises, you actively cultivate a space of awareness and calm within yourself, which can radiate into every aspect of your life. Remember, every step taken in mindfulness is a step toward greater peace and balance.

The simplicity and accessibility of these practices mean they can be seamlessly integrated into your routine, regardless of how busy you might be. Even a few minutes of tai chi in the morning or some gentle yoga poses before bed can make a noticeable difference in how you feel physically and emotionally.

Take control of your mental health by making these activities a regular part of your life. The beauty of mindful movement is that it empowers you to engage directly with your physical and emotional landscapes, teaching resilience and promoting an overall sense of well-being.

Let this chapter remind you that your journey to mindfulness doesn't have to be static or confined to conventional meditation spaces. It can be as dynamic and varied as the movements you explore. You are paving the way to a more serene and joyous life with each mindful step, breath, or stretch.

Start today by choosing one mindful movement activity that resonates with you and commit to integrating it into your day-to-day life. As you do so, observe the subtle yet profound shifts in your stress levels and overall mood. This isn't just about exercise; it's about transforming your everyday experiences into opportunities for growth and peace.

Embrace these practices with an open heart and mind, and watch as they unfold their potential in your life, helping you find calm in the chaos around you.

Chapter 6: Beginning with Mindfulness

"The mind is a powerful instrument. Every thought,

every emotion that you create changes the

chemistry of your body."

Sadhguru

Embrace the Journey: Starting Your Mindfulness Practice

Embarking on the path of mindfulness may initially seem daunting, with its promises of inner peace and heightened awareness. Yet, like any new skill, the key to mastery lies in beginning with small, manageable steps. For those new to mindfulness, understanding where to start is crucial. This chapter will guide you through initiating your practice with straightforward methods that can be seamlessly integrated into your daily routine.

Mindfulness is not about perfection; it's about progression. Starting with simple practices such as mindful breathing or conducting a body scan can significantly ease the entry into mindfulness. These techniques do not require extensive training or special equipment—they can be practiced in the quiet of your home or during a break at work.

The importance of patience and compassion towards oneself cannot be overstressed. Beginners often face frustration when their minds wander frequently during practice. It's vital to approach these moments not as failures but as opportunities to redirect your focus gently. Each return to mindfulness reinforces neural pathways that make future sessions more fruitful.

Finding adequate resources and communities for support is another critical step for beginners. Choose tools that resonate with your learning style and current life situation, whether books, online courses, or local workshops. Engaging with a community or a mentor can also provide encouragement and insights, which are invaluable when starting.

Mindfulness practices are numerous and varied, allowing you to explore and find what works best for you. From meditation apps that guide you through daily practices to journaling exercises that encourage reflection and awareness, tools are abundant at your disposal.

Taking control of your mental space requires active participation in these practices. Rather than passively reading about mindfulness, engaging actively with the techniques taught is crucial. Regular practice builds skill and fosters a habit that can anchor you through life's chaos.

The journey into mindfulness teaches more than just techniques; it opens up a new perspective on stress management and personal growth. As you learn to observe your thoughts without judgment and live more fully in the present moment, you begin to experience the serenity of true emotional mastery.

Remember, starting something new is always challenging, but the rewards of mindfulness are worth the effort. By approaching this practice with an open mind and heart, you set the foundation for a transformative experience that extends beyond stress relief into deep personal insight and peace.

Navigating the start of your mindfulness journey with simple, effective practices can set a solid foundation for beginners. Mindfulness is not about achieving perfection but cultivating awareness and presence in the present moment. Starting with basic techniques like mindful breathing or body scans can help ease beginners into the practice without overwhelming them. These simple practices allow individuals to connect with their bodies and minds, fostering a sense of calm and clarity amidst the chaos of daily life.

Approach mindfulness with curiosity and openness, understanding that it is a skill that improves with practice and patience. As a beginner, it's essential to be gentle with yourself and acknowledge that progress takes time. Patience is key in the mindfulness journey; each moment of practice contributes to personal growth and self-awareness. By embracing a mindset of curiosity and openness, beginners can explore mindfulness without judgment or expectation.

Seeking guidance from mindfulness resources, experienced practitioners, or courses tailored for beginners can provide valuable support. Connecting with a community of like-minded individuals can offer encouragement, accountability, and shared insights. Remember that everyone starts somewhere, and it's okay to be a beginner in mindfulness. Embrace the learning process with an open heart and a willingness to explore new possibilities.

Nurturing Mindfulness as a Beginner

Integrating mindfulness into your daily routine doesn't have to be complicated or time-consuming. By starting with straightforward practices and approaching them with curiosity and patience, beginners can lay a strong foundation for their mindfulness journey. The key is to begin where you are, take small daily steps, and trust in growth and self-discovery. Allow yourself the grace to learn and evolve as you embark toward a more significant presence and inner peace.

As a beginner in mindfulness, it's crucial to acknowledge the significance of patience and self-compassion. The journey into mindfulness is not a race; it's a process that requires gentle persistence and understanding towards oneself. Embracing mindfulness practices can be challenging, especially when faced with the initial hurdles of calming a busy mind or focusing on the present moment. Therefore, it's essential to approach this journey with gentleness and empathy, recognizing that progress takes time and effort.

Practice self-compassion by being kind and understanding towards yourself as you navigate the complexities of mindfulness. It's common to feel frustrated or overwhelmed when thoughts wander during meditation or when emotions seem challenging to manage. Instead of being critical, offer yourself the same kindness you would to a close friend facing similar challenges. Remember that mindfulness is a skill that improves with practice, and setbacks are an inherent part of the learning process.

Cultivate patience as you embark on your mindfulness journey. Understand that change doesn't happen overnight, and taking small steps toward building a consistent practice is okay. Rome wasn't built in a day, and similarly, mastering mindfulness requires dedication and perseverance over time. Be patient with yourself as you learn to observe your thoughts without judgment or explore different techniques to anchor yourself in the present moment.

Remember that progress is not linear in moments of doubt or frustration. There will be days when mindfulness comes effortlessly and others when it feels like an uphill battle. Embrace these fluctuations with an open heart, knowing each experience contributes to your growth and understanding of mindfulness. Remember that every moment spent in awareness is a step forward on your journey toward inner peace and clarity, no matter how brief.

Celebrate small victories along the way. Whether it's managing to stay present for an extra minute during meditation or noticing a pattern in your thoughts, acknowledge these achievements with gratitude and encouragement. By recognizing and appreciating your progress, you reinforce positive habits and motivate yourself to continue exploring the depths of mindfulness.

In times of struggle or impatience, lean on your support system. Connect with other beginners or experienced practitioners who can offer guidance, reassurance, and wisdom from their journeys. Seeking out communities dedicated to mindfulness can provide valuable insights, accountability, and inspiration as you navigate the challenges of starting.

Remember that you are not alone in this endeavor. Countless individuals have walked this path before you, facing unique obstacles and triumphs. By embracing patience and compassion towards yourself as a beginner, you pave the way for a transformative experience filled with growth, self-discovery, and profound inner peace.

As a beginner in the practice of mindfulness, it is essential to find resources and communities that support your journey. Surrounding yourself with like-minded individuals can provide encouragement, guidance, and a sense of belonging as you navigate this new territory. Seek mindfulness groups or classes specifically tailored for beginners, where you can learn from experienced practitioners and connect with others who are also starting their mindfulness path.

Online platforms and apps can be valuable tools for beginners, offering guided meditations, mindfulness exercises, and a wealth of information on incorporating mindfulness into your daily life. Podcasts focused on mindfulness can also be a source of inspiration and knowledge, allowing you to learn from experts in the field and gain insights into different aspects of mindfulness practice.

Books written for beginners by seasoned mindfulness teachers can provide in-depth explanations, practical tips, and step-by-step guidance on cultivating mindfulness. Look for titles that resonate with you and align with your goals for practicing mindfulness. Workshops and retreats offer immersive experiences that can deepen your understanding of mindfulness and provide a supportive environment for growth.

Mindfulness websites often feature articles, videos, and resources catering to beginners, covering basic meditation techniques, mindful breathing exercises, and ways to integrate mindfulness into everyday activities. Social media groups focused on mindfulness can also offer a sense of community and a platform for sharing experiences with fellow beginners.

Remember that finding the right resources and communities is a personal journey, so explore different options to see what resonates with you. It's okay to try various approaches until you find the ones that best support your mindfulness practice.

Embrace this exploration with an open mind and a willingness to learn from diverse sources.

Embarking on a mindfulness journey may initially feel daunting, but starting with simple, effective practices can make it accessible and rewarding. Mindful breathing or body scans are potent pathways to deeper self-awareness and peace. Embrace these tools with the curiosity of a beginner and allow yourself the space to grow.

Patience and compassion towards oneself are indispensable on this path. Remember, learning mindfulness is akin to nurturing a plant; it grows gradually and requires consistent care. Treat yourself as kindly as a friend learning a new skill. This gentle approach will not only make the process enjoyable but also sustainable.

Finding resources and communities for support is crucial. These resources, whether books, online courses, or local groups, can offer guidance and companionship. Engaging with others on this journey can provide motivation and insight, making your practice a personal and shared experience.

By integrating mindfulness into your daily routine, you take an active role in managing stress and enhancing your overall well-being. Each moment of mindfulness adds up, helping you build a resilient and joyful life amidst the chaos. Start small, stay consistent, and watch how these practices transform your perspective and reality.

Let this be your invitation to enter a world where calm prevails over chaos. With each mindful breath, you reclaim a piece of serenity and joy in your life. Remember, every journey begins with a single step—take yours today.

Chapter 7: Alleviating Stress through Awareness

"With mindfulness, you can establish yourself in the

present in order to touch the wonders of life

that are available in that moment."

Thich Nhat Hanh

From Tension to Tranquility: Harnessing Mindfulness to Master Stress

The relentless pace of modern life often leaves many grappling with an overwhelming sense of stress. However, the practice of mindfulness offers a transformative approach to not only manage this stress but to thrive amidst it. By understanding and applying mindfulness techniques, individuals can interrupt the cycle of anxiety, fostering a rejuvenating and sustaining relaxation.

Mindfulness is not just about being aware; it's about actively shifting how we process our experiences. It allows us to step back and observe our thoughts and feelings without judgment, creating a space between stimulus and response. This space is powerful—we can choose how to react rather than being swept away by emotion. Learning this non-reactive stance can be incredibly empowering for anyone struggling with stress.

Rewiring the Stress Response

At its core, mindfulness influences the very architecture of our brains. Research has shown that consistent mindfulness practice can modify neural pathways associated with stress reactivity, enhancing areas linked to awareness, concentration, and emotional regulation. This neuroplasticity suggests that our brain's capacity to adapt is not fixed but rather highly responsive to practices like mindfulness.

The Art of Mindful Stress Reduction

One fundamental aspect of reducing stress through mindfulness involves recognizing when stressors activate our fight-or-flight response. This awareness is critical as it is the first step in choosing a different path that leads to calmness and clarity.

Techniques such as mindful breathing help alleviate immediate stress and condition the mind and body to maintain peace over prolonged periods.

Step Into Calm: A Strategic Approach to Mindfulness

Step 1: Recognize the Signs of Stress

Identify early signs of stress—perhaps a quickened heartbeat or a sudden mood shift. Regular check-ins with your physical and emotional states throughout the day can alert you to rising stress levels before they escalate.

Step 2: Practice Mindful Awareness

When you notice signs of stress, pause. Close your eyes if possible, and direct your attention inward. Focus on your breath and observe any sensations in your body or shifts in your thoughts without attempting to alter them.

Step 3: Cultivate Non-Reactivity

This step involves observing your thoughts and emotions as they are—transient states that do not define you. By distancing yourself from these reactions, you allow them to pass like clouds in the sky, reducing their impact on your mood and behavior.

Step 4: Utilize Mindful Breathing for Stress Reduction

Engage deeply with your breath. Inhale slowly through your nose, letting your abdomen expand fully, then exhale slowly through your mouth. This type of breathing activates the parasympathetic nervous system, promoting a state of calmness.

Step 5: Incorporate Mindfulness Breaks Throughout the Day

Set aside short periods—maybe three to five minutes—several times daily for focused mindfulness exercises like body scans or mini-meditations. These breaks are vital for resetting your stress levels and reinforcing your mindfulness practice.

Step 6: Establish a Mindfulness Toolbox for Stress Management

Create a personalized set of mindfulness tools you can use in stressful situations. This may include recorded guided meditations, written reminders for breath exercises, or playlists of calming music that facilitate relaxation.

By integrating these steps into daily life, mindfulness becomes more than just a practice—it evolves into a way of being. This transformation doesn't happen overnight; it requires consistency and commitment. Yet, each small step contributes to greater emotional resilience and a more profound sense of peace amidst life's chaos.

Harnessing Mindfulness: Techniques for Stress Management

Mindfulness is a powerful tool for managing stress, offering a pathway to interrupt the cycle of anxious thoughts and promote relaxation responses in the body. By cultivating a mindset of non-reactivity, individuals can navigate stressful situations with greater ease and resilience. Mindfulness practice involves being fully present and observing thoughts and feelings without judgment. This awareness allows individuals to respond to stressors more accurately and intentionally rather than impulsively.

One technique to manage stress through mindfulness is to focus on the breath. Paying attention to the inhalation and exhalation can anchor you in the present moment, diverting your mind from worrisome thoughts. When stressful situations arise, take a moment to pause and bring your awareness to your breath. Notice the sensation of air entering and leaving your body, allowing it to calm your mind and center your thoughts.

Body scan exercises are another effective way to cultivate mindfulness and reduce stress. This practice involves systematically bringing attention to different body parts noting any areas of tension or discomfort. Scanning your body with awareness can release physical tension and promote relaxation. Regular body scan exercises can help you become more attuned to bodily sensations and better equipped to manage stress responses.

Mindful observation of thoughts is essential for cultivating non-reactivity. Instead of getting caught up in the content of your thoughts, try observing them as if they were passing clouds in the sky. Notice them without judgment or attachment, allowing them to come and go without getting entangled in their narrative. This practice can help you detach from negative thought patterns and reduce their impact on your emotional well-being.

Unveiling Mindfulness: A Gateway to Reshaping the Brain's Response to Stress

Understanding how mindfulness can alter the brain's response to stress is critical to unlocking its full potential in alleviating the pressures of daily life. Mindfulness practices have been shown to impact the brain profoundly, rewiring it to respond more calmly and rationally to stressors. By engaging in mindfulness regularly, individuals can cultivate a more balanced and harmonious way of being, promoting relaxation responses in the body that counteract the cycle of anxious thoughts.

One crucial aspect of mindfulness is its ability to interrupt the automatic stress response, shifting the focus from reactive thinking to a more present-centered awareness. This shift allows individuals to observe their thoughts and emotions without judgment, creating space for a calmer and more measured response to stressors. By fostering a mindset of non-reactivity and acceptance, mindfulness empowers individuals to navigate challenging situations with greater ease and resilience.

Neuroscience research has shown that mindfulness practices can change the structure and function of the brain. Regular meditation and mindfulness have been linked to increased gray matter density in regions associated with emotion regulation, self-awareness, and perspective-taking. These changes can lead to improved emotional regulation, reduced reactivity to stress, and enhanced overall well-being.

The brain's plasticity allows it to adapt and reorganize in response to experiences, enabling individuals to train their brains through mindfulness practices. By focusing on the present moment and cultivating awareness of thoughts and emotions, individuals can strengthen neural pathways associated with calmness and resilience, gradually reducing the impact of stress on both the mind and body.

Through mindfulness, individuals can learn to respond to stressors from a place of clarity and calm rather than reacting impulsively or emotionally. This shift in perspective not only reduces immediate feelings of anxiety but also has long-term benefits for overall mental health and well-being. By understanding how mindfulness can reshape the brain's response to stress, individuals can harness its transformative power to cultivate a greater sense of peace and serenity.

Framework for Mindfulness Practice in Stress Reduction

The framework for practicing mindfulness exercises tailored for stress reduction is designed to provide a structured approach to managing stress effectively. Following a step-by-step process, individuals can identify stressors, recognize bodily responses, engage in specific mindfulness techniques, and reflect on the outcomes. This iterative model emphasizes the importance of regular practice and adaptation to achieve optimal stress management results.

Identifying Stressors and Body Responses

The initial step involves identifying the sources of stress in one's life. This may include work deadlines, relationship issues, financial concerns, or health-related worries. By pinpointing these stressors, individuals can better understand their triggers and begin to address them proactively. Simultaneously, it is crucial to recognize how the body responds to stress, such as increased heart rate, muscle tension, shallow breathing, or racing thoughts. Heightened awareness of these physical cues can indicate when stress levels are rising.

Mindfulness Techniques for Stress Reduction

Once stressors and body responses are identified, individuals can engage in mindfulness exercises tailored explicitly for stress reduction. These techniques may include:

- Focused Breathing: Concentrating on the breath to calm the mind and body.

- Observing Thoughts without Judgment: Acknowledging thoughts without attaching value or criticism.

- Physical Sensations Meditation: Bringing attention to bodily sensations to ground oneself in the present moment.

Reflection and Adaptation

After practicing mindfulness exercises, reflecting on their effectiveness in mitigating stress is essential. Individuals can evaluate whether the techniques helped reduce anxiety levels, promote relaxation, or enhance emotional regulation. Based on this assessment, adapting one's approach by modifying techniques or exploring new practices that align better with individual needs is crucial. This reflective process allows for continuous improvement in stress management through mindfulness.

Practical Implications and Future Development

By following this framework, individuals can develop a sustainable mindfulness practice that effectively supports stress reduction. The structured approach offers a clear pathway for cultivating resilience and promoting emotional well-being. Moreover, the iterative nature of the model encourages ongoing reflection and adaptation, fostering growth in mindfulness skills over time.

In this chapter, we have explored the profound impact of mindfulness on stress reduction. By embracing mindfulness techniques, you equip yourself with a powerful tool that manages stress and transforms your approach to challenging situations. The ability to cultivate non-reactivity allows you to observe your thoughts and feelings without being overwhelmed, fostering a sense of calm and control.

Understanding how mindfulness reshapes your brain's response to stress is crucial. Regular practice can rewire neural pathways, enhancing resilience and decreasing susceptibility to stress-induced anxiety. This knowledge isn't just empowering—it's a call to action. Integrating mindfulness exercises into your daily routine actively improves mental and emotional health.

Take control of your stress by practicing the mindfulness exercises we discussed. These are designed to fit your busy schedule, offering practical solutions that bring tangible results. Remember, the goal is not to eliminate stress but to change how you interact. Stress doesn't have to be a roadblock; it can lead to personal growth and resilience with the right tools.

Embrace these strategies with confidence, knowing that each step you take is building towards a more balanced and serene life. Your journey towards mastering stress through mindfulness is not just about coping—it's about thriving. Each mindful moment is a step away from chaos and towards reclaiming joy in your life.

Start today. The power to mold your brain's response to stress lies in your hands, and each small practice adds to significant changes. Let these insights guide you as you continue on your path of personal development, equipped with the knowledge that you can transform stress into serenity.

Chapter 8: Enriching Your Practice with Mindfulness Literature

"Mindfulness is the aware, balanced acceptance of the present experience. It isn't more complicated than that."

Sylvia Boorstein

Unlock the Power of Mindfulness Through the Pages of a Book

Mindfulness isn't just a practice; it's a journey that begins with understanding. Finding solace through mindfulness can seem daunting in the bustling world where stress is a constant companion. However, literature on mindfulness offers a gateway to transforming stress into serenity. The right books provide techniques and diverse perspectives that enrich your mindfulness practice. Here lies an opportunity to discover critical works that cater to various interests and needs, from scientific explanations to personal anecdotes and practical exercises.

Integrating mindfulness into your life lies in deepening your understanding of its principles. Each book written about mindfulness serves as a bridge between abstract concepts and tangible practices. By exploring a variety of texts, you are invited into a world where each author's insights add layers to your comprehension of mindfulness. This deepened understanding is crucial for anyone seeking to maintain their center amidst chaos.

Moreover, reading these carefully selected books lets you apply insights directly to your daily routine. Whether you're a busy professional, a parent juggling multiple responsibilities, or someone simply trying to find peace in hectic times, applying learned techniques can significantly enhance your quality of life. Each chapter and each page turn can become a step towards personal growth and emotional mastery.

It's essential to approach this literary journey with an open mind and heart. The diversity in mindfulness literature ensures that there is something relatable for everyone, regardless of their background or current level of practice. From neuroscience-based approaches by authors like Daniel Siegel to the more spiritual perspectives offered by Thich Nhat Hanh, the spectrum is broad yet profoundly interconnected.

Choosing the right books might initially seem overwhelming. Focus on those that resonate with your current situation but also challenge you to explore new dimensions of mindfulness. For instance, if you're grappling with anxiety, books focusing on mindfulness-based stress reduction could offer practical strategies for managing your symptoms. Conversely, if you're interested in the philosophical underpinnings of mindfulness, exploring texts rooted in Buddhist teachings might provide deeper philosophical insights.

Remember that the goal isn't just to read but to transform reading into action. Practical exercises included in many mindfulness books encourage active participation. Engage with these exercises regularly as part of your daily or weekly routine. This active engagement helps cement the concepts learned and makes them more accessible when stress levels rise.

Lastly, remember that this literary journey is also about personal connection. As you read stories and insights from authors who have navigated their paths through chaos to calmness, you'll likely see reflections of your struggles and triumphs. This connection not only humanizes the practice of mindfulness but also reinforces the idea that you are not alone in your quest for peace.

By embracing the wisdom in these pages, you empower yourself with knowledge and practical tools that pave the way toward a centered and joyful life—even amidst inevitable turmoil.

In mindfulness literature, a treasure trove of wisdom is waiting to be explored. These books cater to diverse interests and needs, offering valuable insights, practical techniques, and varied perspectives on incorporating mindfulness into daily life. Whether you are seeking to understand the science behind mindfulness, looking for practical exercises to implement, or hoping to gain real-life applications of mindfulness practices, there is a book for you.

The best mindfulness books guide the journey to self-discovery and personal growth. They offer a roadmap to navigate the complexities of our minds and emotions, providing tools to cultivate inner peace and resilience in the face of life's challenges. By delving into these books, readers can deepen their understanding of mindfulness practices and uncover new ways to enhance their well-being.

One key benefit of exploring mindfulness literature is the opportunity to learn from experts in the field who have dedicated their lives to studying and practicing mindfulness. These authors share their knowledge, experiences, and insights with readers, offering guidance on effectively integrating mindfulness into everyday routines. By immersing oneself in the wisdom contained within these pages, one can gain a deeper appreciation for the transformative power of mindfulness in fostering emotional balance and mental clarity.

Mindfulness books provide a space for reflection and introspection, allowing readers to pause and contemplate their thoughts, feelings, and actions. They encourage self-awareness and self-compassion, guiding individuals to understand themselves and others better. Through engaging with these texts, readers can develop a greater sense of empathy, connection, and presence in their interactions with the world around them.

Exploring various mindfulness books can spark inspiration and motivation for personal growth and development. Each book offers a unique perspective on mindfulness, shedding light on different aspects of the practice and its applications in daily life. By incorporating insights from multiple sources, readers can enrich their understanding of mindfulness and tailor their training to suit their needs and preferences.

As you embark on this journey through mindfulness literature, remember that each book has something valuable. Whether you are drawn to scientific explanations, practical exercises, or personal anecdotes, there is a book that will resonate with you. Exploring different titles and authors can expand your knowledge base, deepen your practice, and evolve toward greater peace and well-being.

Exploring Mindfulness Through Literature

Reading various mindfulness books can provide valuable insights, techniques, and perspectives on incorporating mindfulness into one's life. A deepening understanding of mindfulness practices through diverse literary perspectives offers a unique opportunity to explore different approaches and applications of mindfulness. By delving into various books on mindfulness, readers can gain a richer understanding of the practice and its benefits, ultimately enhancing their personal growth and development.

One key benefit of exploring different mindfulness books is the exposure to various perspectives and insights. Each author brings unique experiences and expertise, offering readers diverse tools and techniques to incorporate into their practice. By immersing oneself in various mindfulness literature, individuals can expand their knowledge base and discover new ways to approach challenges and obstacles with a mindful mindset.

Another advantage of engaging with mindfulness books is the opportunity to deepen one's understanding of mindfulness practices' underlying principles and science. By exploring different texts, readers can better understand how mindfulness affects the brain, body, and overall well-being. This deeper understanding can empower individuals to tailor their practice to suit their needs and goals effectively.

Moreover, diverse mindfulness literature can offer practical exercises and real-life applications that resonate with readers personally. By experimenting with the exercises and techniques outlined in various books, individuals can discover which methods work best for them and integrate them seamlessly into their daily routines. This hands-on approach allows for a more immersive experience with mindfulness, leading to tangible results and lasting change.

Incorporating insights from mindfulness literature can also

inspire ongoing personal growth and development. By learning from different authors and experts in the field, individuals can continue to evolve their practice and deepen their connection with themselves and the world around them. This continuous learning fosters curiosity, openness, and receptivity to new ideas and experiences.

Overall, exploring diverse literary perspectives on mindfulness enriches one's practice by offering fresh insights, practical tools, and inspirational guidance. Individuals can deepen their understanding of the practice by engaging with various mindfulness books, refine their skills, and cultivate a greater sense of inner peace and well-being. By embracing this journey of exploration and discovery through literature, readers can enhance their personal growth and profoundly transform their lives.

Applying the insights gained from mindfulness literature can significantly enhance your practice and overall growth. By delving into the wisdom shared in these books, you can deepen your understanding of mindfulness and cultivate a more profound connection with yourself and the world around you. One key aspect of applying these insights is consistency. Consistently practicing mindfulness techniques and integrating the teachings from these books into your daily life is crucial for experiencing lasting benefits.

Mindfulness literature can guide you, offering practical strategies and tools to implement in your daily routine. As you read through various mindfulness books, take note of the exercises, meditations, or reflections shared by the authors. Choose a few practices that resonate with you and commit to incorporating them into your day-to-day life. Whether it's a simple breathing exercise, a gratitude journaling practice, or mindful walking, these techniques can help you stay grounded and present amidst life's challenges.

Another way to apply insights from mindfulness literature is through self-reflection. Consider the concepts presented in the books you read and how they relate to your experiences. Journaling can be a powerful tool for processing your thoughts and emotions, allowing you to gain clarity and insight into your inner workings. By reflecting on what resonates with you and what areas you struggle with, you can tailor your mindfulness practice to suit your unique needs.

Integrating mindfulness into different aspects of your life is also essential for personal growth. As you apply the insights from mindfulness literature, consider how you can bring mindfulness into your relationships, work environment, and daily interactions. Practice active listening during conversations, cultivate compassion towards others, and approach challenges calmly and intently. You can foster a sense of balance and well-being by infusing mindfulness into all areas of your life.

Embracing a beginner's mindset is critical when applying insights from mindfulness literature. Approach each practice with openness and curiosity, allowing yourself to learn and grow. Remember that progress takes time, and it's okay to encounter setbacks or challenges on your journey towards greater mindfulness. Stay patient with yourself and trust in the process of personal development.

Lastly, remember that self-compassion is an integral part of mindfulness practice. Be kind to yourself as you navigate this path of self-discovery and growth. Acknowledge your efforts and celebrate small victories along the way. Treating yourself with compassion creates a nurturing environment for personal transformation to unfold.

Incorporating the wisdom found in mindfulness literature into your daily life can lead to profound shifts in how you perceive yourself and the world around you. Stay committed to your practice, remain open to new insights, and embrace each moment with awareness and presence. As you continue this journey of self-discovery through mindfulness, remember that every step forward is a step towards greater peace, resilience, and joy in your life.

As we journey through the ever-evolving landscape of mindfulness, the books highlighted in this chapter serve as guides and companions for deeper awareness and personal growth. Each book offers unique insights and practical strategies crucial for enhancing their mindfulness practice. Whether you're a beginner or well-versed in mindfulness, these literary resources cater to a spectrum of needs and preferences, ensuring something valuable for every reader.

The diversity of perspectives presented through these texts enriches your understanding of mindfulness, providing a broader context and more profound comprehension of its principles. This variety allows you to explore multiple facets of mindfulness, from scientific explanations to experiential anecdotes, helping you grasp the concept holistically. It's imperative to remember that integrating these insights into your daily routine can significantly amplify your personal development and emotional resilience.

Applying what you've learned from these books can be transformative. Start by incorporating one or two techniques into your daily life and gradually expand as you feel more comfortable. The practical applications discussed are designed to fit seamlessly into your busy schedule, making it feasible to maintain consistency in your practice. Remember, consistency is critical when reaping the benefits of mindfulness.

Lastly, empower yourself with the knowledge that you have the innate ability to manage stress and enhance your wellbeing through mindfulness. These books are tools that equip you with the skills to navigate life's challenges more effectively. Embrace this journey with an open mind and a willing heart, knowing each step forward is a move towards a more centered and joyful life.

Engage actively with these resources and let them inspire you towards greater peace and understanding. The path to mastering mindfulness is rewarding and profound—embrace it fully for all the serenity and joy it brings into your life.

Chapter 9: The Art of Everyday Mindfulness

"The art of peaceful living comes down to living

compassionately & wisely."

Allan Lokos

Unlock the Power of the Present Moment

Mindfulness isn't just a retreat from the chaos; it's a practical skill that can be woven into the fabric of our everyday lives. The essence of mindfulness lies in its simplicity and universal applicability, which can transform mundane interactions into moments of deep presence and connection. This chapter delves into how integrating mindfulness into daily routines enhances awareness and cultivates resilience and gratitude amidst life's inevitable turbulence.

For many, mindfulness conjures images of lengthy meditation sessions or extended periods of solitude. However, the true power of mindfulness is realized when it becomes part of our routine activities. By learning to apply mindfulness in ordinary tasks such as eating, walking, or even during conversations, we develop a continuous state of awareness that helps us break free from autopilot mode. This heightened awareness allows us to savor every moment and react more thoughtfully to the world.

Experimenting with simple mindfulness techniques that can seamlessly fit into a busy schedule is crucial. Techniques such as mindful breathing or focused attention can be practiced while performing daily chores or during short breaks at work. These practices do not require extra time; instead, they transform the quality of time we already have. Through consistent practice, these techniques help stabilize our minds and clarify our thoughts and emotions.

Recognizing opportunities for mindfulness in everyday interactions and emotional responses is another vital skill. It involves being fully present during conversations, listening actively without judgment, and observing our emotional reactions without being overwhelmed. This improves our relationships and provides deep insights into our emotional patterns, fostering emotional intelligence and resilience.

Moreover, integrating mindfulness helps develop a compassionate attitude towards oneself and others. It encourages us to accept our experiences without resistance, reducing stress and enhancing our capacity to deal with challenges more gracefully. This compassionate approach is particularly beneficial in managing the high-pressure situations that often characterize modern life.

To make these practices more accessible, it's essential to start small with what feels manageable and gradually build on those experiences. Whether dedicating five minutes to observe your breath each morning or walking mindfully between meetings at work, each small step contributes to a more significant transformation.

Lastly, embracing mindfulness in daily life isn't just about personal peace; it's about creating ripples of calmness around us. As we become more present and centered, our interactions naturally become more genuine and empathetic, influencing others positively. This interconnectedness underscores the personal benefits of mindfulness and its potential to foster a kinder, more conscious society.

By embracing these practices with an open heart and mind, you empower yourself to navigate life's complexities with greater ease and joy. Start where you are, use what you have, and do what you can—this is the essence of everyday mindfulness that leads to lasting change.

Finding moments of peace and presence can feel like an unattainable luxury in the hustle and bustle of our daily lives. Yet, integrating mindfulness into our ordinary activities can transform these mundane moments into opportunities for deep connection and awareness. Mindfulness in everyday life is not reserved for special occasions or lengthy meditation sessions; it is a practice that can be seamlessly woven into the fabric of our daily routines. By bringing a conscious awareness to even the most routine tasks, we can cultivate a continuous state of mindfulness that enriches our experiences and nurtures our well-being.

Mindfulness is not about adding more tasks to our overflowing to-do lists; it is about infusing intention and attention into activities we already engage in. Whether washing dishes, walking the dog, or sipping a cup of tea, each moment presents a chance to be fully present and engaged. Approaching these activities with mindfulness allows us to break free from autopilot mode and truly savor the richness of each experience.

One way to bring mindfulness into ordinary activities is by focusing on the sensations present in the moment. As you go about your day, pay attention to the sights, sounds, smells, tastes, and textures surrounding you. Engage your senses fully, immersing yourself in the present moment without judgment or distraction. This simple practice can help anchor you in the now and foster a deeper connection with your surroundings.

Another effective way to cultivate mindfulness in everyday activities is by incorporating intentional pauses throughout your day. Instead of rushing from one task to the next, take a few moments to pause, breathe, and center yourself before transitioning. These pauses act as checkpoints that allow you to reset and refocus your attention on the present moment. Whether it's a brief moment of stillness before answering an email or taking a mindful breath before starting a new task, these pauses can help ground you in the here and now.

By infusing mindfulness into ordinary activities, we enhance our presence and cultivate a greater sense of gratitude and interconnectedness with ourselves and the world around us. Each moment becomes an opportunity for growth, reflection, and connection—a chance to experience life more fully and deeply. Embrace the power of mindfulness in your everyday life and discover the profound impact it can have on your well-being and overall sense of fulfillment.

Integrating Mindfulness into Daily Life

Experimenting with mindfulness techniques that seamlessly fit into your daily routine can be a transformative experience. You can cultivate a heightened awareness and presence by incorporating simple practices into your everyday life. One effective technique is mindful breathing. Please take a few moments throughout your day to focus on your breath, noticing its rhythm and how it feels as it enters and leaves your body. This practice can anchor you to the present moment, helping to alleviate stress and promote calmness.

Another technique that can be effortlessly integrated into your daily life is mindful eating. Before each meal or snack, take a moment to appreciate the food before you. Notice the colors, textures, and smells. Eat slowly and savor each bite, paying attention to the flavors and sensations in your mouth. This practice enhances your enjoyment of food and encourages mindful consumption and healthy eating habits.

Mindful walking is another powerful technique that can be practiced during daily strolls or commutes. As you walk, focus on the sensation of each step touching the ground. Notice the movement of your body, the sounds around you, and the sights you encounter. Walking mindfully can help ground you in the present moment and foster a deep connection with your surroundings.

Incorporating mindful pauses throughout your day can also significantly impact your overall well-being. Set aside a few moments at regular intervals to pause, breathe, and check in with yourself. Use these pauses as opportunities to recenter and realign with your intentions for the day. By taking these short breaks, you can prevent overwhelm and cultivate a sense of clarity and focus.

Practicing gratitude is another simple yet powerful way to infuse mindfulness into your daily life. At the end of each day, take a moment to reflect on three things you are grateful for. This practice shifts your focus from what is lacking to what is abundant in your life, fostering a positive outlook and increasing feelings of contentment.

Engaging in mindful listening during conversations is an excellent way to deepen your connections and enhance communication. Practice active listening by giving your full attention to the speaker without formulating responses. Truly listen to their words, tone, and body language, fostering empathy and understanding in your interactions.

By experimenting with these mindfulness techniques in various aspects of your daily life, you can gradually cultivate a more conscious and intentional way of living. Each practice offers a unique opportunity to enhance self-awareness, reduce stress, and nurture a deeper connection with yourself and those around you. Start small, be consistent, and allow yourself to fully immerse in the present moment through these simple yet impactful practices.

In our daily lives, opportunities for mindfulness are abundant, waiting to be recognized and embraced. Interactions with others and our emotional responses are fertile grounds for practicing mindfulness. By cultivating awareness in these moments, we can deepen our connections with ourselves and those around us. When engaging in conversations, be present. Listen actively without formulating your response while the other person is speaking. Notice the tone of their voice, their body language, and the emotions behind their words. This practice not only enhances communication but also fosters empathy and understanding.

Emotional responses often occur automatically, triggered by past experiences or conditioned patterns. Mindfulness invites us to pause before reacting, creating a space for conscious choices rather than habitual responses. When faced with a challenging situation, take a moment to breathe deeply and observe the emotions arising within you. Acknowledge these feelings without judgment, allowing them to exist without being consumed by them. This simple act of awareness can prevent impulsive reactions and promote emotional intelligence.

In conflict or disagreement, mindfulness can act as a bridge to compassion. Instead of escalating tension, pause to consider the other person's perspective. Empathy arises naturally when we step into someone else's shoes, recognizing their humanity and vulnerabilities. We nurture harmony and connection in our relationships by responding from a place of understanding rather than defensiveness.

Self-awareness is at the core of mindful interactions. Before projecting our emotions onto others, we must recognize and validate our feelings first. Take time to check in with yourself throughout the day. Notice any signs of stress or unease in your body and mind. By acknowledging your inner state, you can respond more authentically in your interactions, fostering genuine connections based on transparency and openness.

Every interaction is an opportunity for growth through mindfulness. Whether a brief conversation with a colleague or a heartfelt exchange with a loved one, each moment holds the potential for deeper understanding. By bringing conscious awareness to these encounters, we enrich our relationships and cultivate a sense of harmony within ourselves and the world around us.

Mindfulness in interactions and emotional responses empowers us to navigate life's complexities gracefully. Through conscious presence and compassionate understanding, we can transform conflicts into opportunities for connection and personal growth. By recognizing the inherent value of each moment, we embrace the beauty of human relationships and the richness they bring to our lives.

Mindfulness isn't just a practice for serene moments of meditation; it is a vibrant, practical approach to enriching the textures of everyday life. Integrating mindful awareness into routine activities enhances your presence and cultivates a deeper connection with the world around you. This continuous state of awareness helps break the cycle of automatic, non-conscious behavior, allowing you to live more fully in each moment.

Experimenting with mindfulness techniques that fit seamlessly into your daily schedule can transform mundane tasks into opportunities for growth and reflection. Whether through mindful eating, conscious breathing during brief work breaks, or attentive listening in conversations, each action offers a chance to slow down and appreciate the nuances of the present.

Moreover, interactions and emotional responses provide fertile ground for practicing mindfulness. Recognizing these opportunities allows you to respond more thoughtfully to life's challenges. Embracing this approach reduces stress and bolsters resilience, making you better equipped to handle adversity gracefully.

Remember, every step taken in mindfulness is a step toward reclaiming joy and serenity in your life. Start small if needed; even a few minutes of mindful breathing daily can significantly impact your well-being. Encourage yourself to be patient and persistent because the benefits of mindfulness unfold gradually and beautifully.

Embrace these practices with an open heart and mind, and watch as they bring a profound sense of calm and clarity into your chaos. As you continue on this journey, know that you are cultivating a skill and a way of being that resonates with peace and joy deep within.

Chapter 10: Mindfulness as Therapy

"Training your mind to be in the present

moment is the #1 key to making

healthier choices."

Susan Albers

Unveiling the Power of Mindfulness in Modern Therapy

In today's fast-paced world, where stress and anxiety frequently overwhelm us, finding effective strategies to manage mental health has become crucial. Mindfulness therapy techniques offer a promising approach, blending traditional psychotherapeutic methods with the ancient practice of mindfulness. This fusion provides a powerful toolkit for addressing common psychological issues such as anxiety, depression, and chronic stress, especially pertinent for those feeling lost in the chaos of daily responsibilities.

Mindfulness therapy is not just about sitting quietly; it actively engages with one's mental processes. It helps individuals observe their thoughts and feelings without judgment, providing a unique way to manage emotional upheavals. By incorporating mindfulness into therapeutic practices, people can better understand their emotional triggers and construct healthier coping mechanisms.

The synergy between psychotherapy and mindfulness can be particularly transformative. Traditional psychotherapy often focuses on exploring past traumas and understanding personality constructs, while mindfulness encourages living in the present moment and observing one's current experiences. This combination allows for a holistic treatment approach, enabling individuals to heal from past wounds while cultivating resilience against future stressors.

For those new to this concept, applying mindfulness strategies might seem daunting. However, it involves straightforward practices like guided meditations, breathing exercises, and body scans. These methods do not require special equipment or extensive training; they are accessible tools that can be integrated into daily routines to foster significant improvements in mental health.

Individuals need to recognize that they possess the innate ability to influence their mental states positively. Mindfulness therapy empowers people by showing them that they have control over their responses to external circumstances. This realization is vital in transforming stress into serenity and reclaiming joy in life.

Implementing these techniques requires consistency and patience. Mastering mindfulness takes time, as one would not expect to play a musical instrument perfectly without practice. Starting with small steps, like dedicating a few minutes each day to meditation, can lead to profound changes over time.

By embracing mindfulness therapy techniques, individuals not only improve their mental health but also enhance their overall quality of life. They learn to stay grounded amid chaos, making mindful living not just a therapy form but a lifestyle choice that promotes lasting well-being.

In this context, understanding and applying the principles of mindfulness in therapy is more than just learning how to cope; it's about transforming one's life by developing a deep-seated sense of peace and fulfillment amidst everyday challenges.

Mindfulness therapy techniques offer a practical and effective approach to managing mental health issues such as anxiety and depression. By blending traditional psychotherapy with mindfulness practices, individuals can gain valuable tools to navigate their emotional challenges. These techniques provide structured exercises, guided meditations, and practical strategies for applying mindfulness in therapeutic contexts, fostering emotional healing and well-being.

Mindfulness practices can help individuals cultivate awareness and presence in the moment, allowing them to observe their thoughts and feelings without judgment. This non-judgmental awareness can be particularly beneficial for those struggling with anxiety or depression, as it can help break the cycle of negative thinking patterns that often accompany these conditions. Through mindfulness therapy, individuals can learn to respond to their emotions with greater clarity and compassion rather than reacting impulsively or getting caught up in harmful thought patterns.

One of the key benefits of mindfulness therapy is its focus on the present moment. Many mental health issues stem from dwelling on the past or worrying about the future, leading to increased stress and anxiety. Mindfulness techniques encourage individuals to anchor themselves in the present moment, helping them let go of rumination and excessive worry. This shift in focus can be transformative, offering relief from the constant cycle of negative thoughts that often accompany anxiety and depression.

Moreover, mindfulness therapy emphasizes self-compassion. Many individuals struggling with mental health issues are overly critical of themselves, which can exacerbate their symptoms. Through mindfulness practices, individuals learn to treat themselves with kindness and understanding, fostering a sense of inner peace and acceptance. This self-compassionate approach can be incredibly healing, allowing individuals to break free from self-destructive thinking and behavior patterns.

Understanding the Synergy Between Psychotherapeutic Approaches and Mindfulness Practices

Combining psychotherapeutic techniques with mindfulness practices in mental health and well-being opens a gateway to profound healing and self-discovery. The amalgamation of these two approaches creates a holistic framework that addresses symptoms of psychological distress and its root causes. Psychotherapy provides a structured foundation for exploring one's thoughts, emotions, and behaviors, while mindfulness offers a gentle yet powerful tool for cultivating awareness and acceptance in the present moment.

By integrating psychotherapeutic principles with mindfulness practices, individuals can delve deep into their inner landscapes, unraveling the complexities of their minds with compassion and curiosity. This synergistic approach encourages individuals to observe their thoughts without judgment, fostering a sense of detachment from self-defeating patterns and beliefs. Through therapy, individuals can gain insights into the underlying issues contributing to their mental health challenges. At the same time, mindfulness equips them with the skills to navigate these inner terrains with grace and resilience.

Psychotherapy often focuses on cognitive restructuring, helping individuals reframe negative thought patterns and cultivate healthier beliefs about themselves and their experiences. When combined with mindfulness practices, this cognitive reshaping becomes even more potent as individuals learn to observe their thoughts from a place of non-judgmental awareness. This dual approach empowers individuals to challenge unhelpful beliefs, release emotional baggage, and embrace a more compassionate view of themselves and others.

Moreover, integrating mindfulness techniques into psychotherapy sessions can enhance emotional regulation and stress management. Mindfulness practices like deep breathing exercises or body scans can help individuals ground themselves in the present moment, allowing them to navigate intense emotions with calmness and clarity. This integration fosters a deeper connection between mind and body, promoting inner balance and emotional well-being.

Ultimately, the synergy between psychotherapeutic approaches and mindfulness practices offers a comprehensive path toward healing, enabling individuals to cultivate self-awareness, emotional resilience, and inner peace. Through this integrated approach, individuals can embark on a transformative journey toward mental wellness, nurturing a harmonious relationship between their thoughts, emotions, and actions.

This fusion of therapeutic modalities provides a multifaceted toolkit for navigating the complexities of the human psyche, offering individuals practical strategies for managing stress, anxiety, depression, and other mental health challenges. As readers explore this integrated approach, they are encouraged to embrace their inherent capacity for growth, self-discovery, and emotional healing, empowering them to reclaim agency over their mental well-being.

As you apply mindfulness strategies for emotional healing and mental health improvement, remember that the key lies in consistent practice and gentle self-exploration. Start by carving out a few daily moments to engage in mindfulness exercises. These can be as simple as focusing on your breath for a few minutes or practicing body scan meditations to tune into physical sensations. By making these practices a part of your daily routine, you gradually build resilience and emotional awareness.

Embrace self-compassion as you navigate your inner landscape. Understand that healing is a process, and it's okay to have setbacks or difficult days. Treat yourself with the kindness you would offer a close friend facing challenges. Acknowledge your emotions without judgment, allowing them to surface and dissipate naturally.

Incorporate mindfulness into daily activities, such as mindful eating or walking. Pay attention to the sensations, sounds, and sights around you as you engage in these tasks. This simple act of presence can ground you in the moment and reduce feelings of overwhelm or anxiety.

Practice gratitude regularly by reflecting on moments of joy or appreciation. Gratitude can shift your focus from what is lacking to what is abundant, fostering a sense of contentment and well-being.

Engage in loving-kindness meditations to cultivate feelings of compassion towards yourself and others. By extending goodwill and kindness towards all beings, including yourself, you nurture a sense of connection and empathy that can be profoundly healing.

Seek support when needed, whether through therapy, support groups, or trusted friends and family members. Opening up about your struggles can alleviate feelings of isolation and provide valuable insights and perspectives on your journey toward emotional healing.

Set realistic goals for yourself, celebrating small victories along the way. Remember that progress is not always linear, and growth often occurs in moments of challenge or discomfort.

Incorporating these mindfulness strategies into your daily life will pave the way for emotional healing, resilience, and improved mental health. Stay committed to your well-being, knowing that every moment of presence and self-compassion contributes to your growth and flourishing.

Mindfulness therapy techniques have proven their worth as powerful allies in the journey toward mental wellness. By integrating traditional psychotherapy with mindfulness practices, these techniques equip you with practical tools to manage conditions like anxiety and depression. This dual approach addresses symptoms and fosters a deeper understanding of your emotional landscape, empowering you to enact lasting change.

Emotional healing is within reach when you apply mindfulness strategies. These practices are more than temporary fixes; they offer a pathway to transform your daily experiences by enhancing emotional resilience. The synergy between psychotherapeutic approaches and mindfulness creates a holistic treatment model that supports sustained mental health improvements.

Taking control of your mental well-being is an active process. Mindfulness practices allow you to cultivate a centered state of mind, even amidst life's chaos. Each strategy discussed provides practical steps that can be seamlessly incorporated into your routine, ensuring that you can maintain progress on your terms.

The key to successfully implementing these techniques lies in consistent practice and dedication. Remember, small, consistent steps lead to significant changes over time. As you continue to apply these mindfulness strategies, you'll likely notice a shift in how you respond to stress and emotional challenges—signaling improvement and transformation.

By embracing mindfulness as a therapeutic tool, you take a decisive step towards reclaiming joy and serenity. This approach isn't just about coping with the present; it's about building a foundation for lasting mental health and well-being. So, let each moment of mindfulness practice be a stepping stone towards a calmer, more centered you. Your journey towards emotional mastery is well underway—keep moving forward with confidence and clarity.

Chapter 11: Digitally Detoxing with Mindfulness

"If you want to conquer the anxiety

of life, live in the moment,

live in the breath."

Amit Ray

Is Your Smartphone Stealing Your Peace?

In today's hyper-connected world, the boundary between online and offline life blurs, often bringing a mix of convenience and chaos. It's easy to fall into the trap of constant connectivity, where every notification pulls you away from moments of peace. Acknowledging the impact of technology on mindfulness and well-being is the first step toward reclaiming your mental space. You are not alone if you feel overwhelmed by digital demands; it's a shared challenge requiring mindful strategies.

The pervasive use of digital devices can lead to a scattered mind, increased stress, and diminished capacity for deep focus. Yet, these tools are integral to modern life, making simply discarding them impractical. Instead, developing strategies for mindful use of digital devices enables you to harness technology's benefits while minimizing disruptions. This approach isn't about shunning technology but integrating it into your life more thoughtfully.

Creating a balance is essential. Finding harmony between digital connectivity and present-moment living doesn't mean drastic changes overnight. It involves small, sustainable shifts that gradually enhance your quality of life. For instance, setting specific times to check emails or social media can significantly reduce stress and increase productivity and presence.

Imagine how much more you could enjoy daily experiences if you were fully present for them rather than thinking about the unread messages on your phone. Mindful practices like scheduled digital detoxes or mindfulness exercises before starting your online sessions can create buffer zones, helping you manage your digital engagements without feeling overwhelmed.

These strategies empower you to control your interactions with technology rather than being controlled by it. They help cultivate a sense of agency over where and how you allocate your attention. You reclaim command over your mental environment by consciously deciding when and where to engage with digital devices.

This empowerment enhances well-being as you learn to prioritize real-world interactions and internal peace over digital disturbances. The benefits extend beyond individual moments, influencing overall life satisfaction and emotional health.

Remember, adopting these practices is a journey that begins with a single step: decide to be present. From there, each small choice builds on the last, creating a more mindful and fulfilling interaction with the digital world around you. Through this chapter's guidance and practical tips, begin this transformative journey towards a balanced life where technology serves you, not the other way around.

In today's fast-paced digital world, it's essential to acknowledge the profound impact that technology can have on our mindfulness and overall well-being. The constant barrage of notifications, emails, and social media updates can lead to perpetual distraction, making staying present in the moment challenging. Our digital devices, while incredibly useful, can also be a double-edged sword, disrupting our ability to focus, relax, and connect with ourselves and others.

Research has shown that excessive screen time can contribute to increased stress levels, decreased attention span, and disrupted sleep patterns. Recognizing the negative consequences of unchecked technology use on our mental and emotional health is crucial. By acknowledging how our devices can impact our well-being, we can begin to take steps toward cultivating a more mindful relationship with technology.

One key strategy for reclaiming mindfulness in a tech-saturated world is setting boundaries around device usage. This could involve establishing specific times during the day when you disconnect from screens, such as during meals or before bedtime. Creating designated tech-free zones in your home, like the bedroom or dining area, can also help promote a sense of calm and presence in your daily life. By consciously choosing when and how you engage with technology, you regain control over its influence on your mental state.

Digital content consumption is another essential practice for fostering mindfulness in the digital age. Before mindlessly scrolling through social media feeds or diving into a binge-watching session, take a moment to pause and ask yourself if this activity aligns with your values and intentions. By approaching digital consumption with awareness and intention, you can avoid falling into patterns of passive consumption that drain your energy and distract you from what truly matters.

Navigating Digital Overload with Mindful Strategies

Digital devices have become integral to our daily lives in today's fast-paced world. From smartphones to laptops, we are constantly connected and bombarded with information. While these devices offer convenience and efficiency, they can also distract and overwhelm us, hindering our ability to be present and mindful. Developing strategies for consciously using digital devices is essential in reclaiming our focus and finding balance in our lives.

Set Boundaries: One effective strategy is establishing clear boundaries with your digital devices. This can include designating specific times for checking emails or social media, turning off notifications during certain hours, or creating tech-free zones in your home. By setting boundaries, you make space for mindfulness and reduce the constant urge to be connected.

Practice Digital Detox: Regularly engaging in digital detoxes can help reset your relationship with technology. This could involve taking a day off from screens, going on a weekend getaway without devices, or participating in activities that do not include technology. Disconnecting from your devices allows you to reconnect with yourself and the world.

Mindful Consumption: When using digital devices, practice mindful consumption by being intentional about what you engage with online. Consciously choose content that uplifts and inspires you rather than feeds into negative emotions or distractions. Be aware of how specific content makes you feel and adjust your consumption accordingly.

Mindful Tech Use: Incorporate mindfulness practices into your use of technology. Before picking up your phone or logging onto a computer, take a moment to check in with yourself. Ask yourself why you are reaching for the device and if there are healthier ways to meet that need. You can make more conscious choices by bringing awareness to your tech habits.

Create Tech-Free Rituals: Integrate tech-free rituals into your daily routine to promote mindfulness and presence. This could include starting your day with a few minutes of meditation instead of scrolling through social media, having device-free meals with loved ones, or winding down in the evening with a book instead of screen time. These rituals help cultivate moments of peace and connection without the constant presence of digital distractions.

Embrace Mindful Communication: When communicating digitally, practice mindful and compassionate communication. Take the time to craft thoughtful responses instead of reacting impulsively. Pause before sending messages or engaging in online discussions, ensuring your words align with your values and intentions.

Reflect Regularly: Lastly, reflect on your relationship with technology regularly. Notice how it impacts your mood, productivity, and overall well-being. Adjust your habits to ensure your digital use aligns with your values and supports your mental health.

By implementing these strategies for mindful use of digital devices, you can cultivate a healthier relationship with technology and create space for mindfulness in your daily life. Remember that you have the power to choose how you engage with digital devices and can prioritize presence and well-being in a tech-saturated world.

In today's fast-paced digital world, finding a balance between staying connected and being present in the moment can be challenging. The constant notifications, emails, and social media updates can easily pull us away from the beauty of the present. However, creating a harmonious relationship between digital connectivity and present-moment living is possible with mindful awareness and intentional choices.

Acknowledge the Impact

Before diving into strategies for balancing digital usage with mindfulness, it's crucial to acknowledge technology's impact on our well-being. Constant exposure to screens can lead to increased stress, decreased focus, and disrupted sleep patterns. Recognizing these effects allows us to take proactive steps toward a healthier relationship with technology.

Develop Mindful Strategies

One effective way to cultivate mindfulness in the digital age is to set boundaries around device usage. Designate specific times of the day for checking emails or social media, allowing for uninterrupted periods of focus on tasks or quality time with loved ones. Practice mindful breathing exercises before engaging with screens, grounding yourself in the present moment and fostering awareness of your intentions.

Establish Tech-Free Zones

Creating designated tech-free zones in your home can help promote presence and connection with those around you. Designate areas like the dining table or bedroom as screen-free spaces, encouraging meaningful conversations and relaxation without digital distractions. Engage in activities that don't involve screens, such as reading a physical book, going for a walk, or practicing yoga, to nurture a sense of balance and well-being.

Embrace Digital Detox Days

Periodically disconnecting from all digital devices can rejuvenate both the mind and body. Plan regular digital detox days, where you engage in offline activities that bring you joy and relaxation. Use this time to connect with nature, engage in creative pursuits, or rest and recharge without the constant stimulation of screens.

Cultivate Mindful Consumption

When using digital devices, practice mindful consumption by being intentional about what you engage with online. Curate your social media feeds to include content that uplifts and inspires you, unfollowing accounts that contribute to negativity or comparison. Set time limits for screen usage and prioritize activities that align with your values and well-being.

Prioritize Human Connection

While digital connectivity has benefits, nothing can replace the depth of human connection experienced in face-to-face interactions. Make time for meaningful conversations with loved ones, putting away devices to fully engage and listen. Practice active listening when communicating digitally, showing empathy and understanding through your responses.

Find Joy in Simple Moments

Incorporate mindfulness practices into your daily routine by savoring simple moments of joy and gratitude. Take time to appreciate nature's beauty, savoring the sights, sounds, and sensations around you. Practice gratitude for the blessings in your life, fostering a positive outlook and cultivating inner peace amidst life's challenges.

Integrating these strategies into your daily life allows you to navigate the digital landscape with greater awareness and intentionality while nurturing a deeper connection with yourself and those around you. Remember that finding balance is an ongoing journey, requiring patience, self-compassion, and a commitment to prioritizing your well-being amidst the noise of modern technology.

Embrace Your Power Over Technology

The influence of technology on our daily lives is undeniable, yet it's crucial to remember that you have the power to manage this impact. Acknowledging how digital devices can affect your mindfulness and well-being, you take the first step toward regaining control. It's about making conscious choices rather than letting habits dictate your life.

Strategies for Mindful Engagement

Developing practical strategies is critical to navigating the digital world without losing touch with your inner self. Setting specific times to check emails or social media can drastically reduce stress and increase your presence in real-world activities. Remember, every small step towards mindful use is a leap towards a more balanced life.

Living in the Present Moment

Creating a balance between online connectivity and living in the moment isn't just beneficial; it's necessary for your mental health and overall happiness. Emphasize face-to-face interactions and immerse yourself in your immediate environment. Let these experiences enrich your life beyond the digital realm.

By actively engaging with technology mindfully, you enhance your well-being and set a positive example for those around you.

Start today because every moment is an opportunity to live more fully, free from the unnecessary distractions that technology can bring.

Chapter 12: Creating Sacred Spaces for Mindfulness

"When you realize nothing is lacking, the

whole world belongs to you."

Lao Tzu

Transform Your Space, Transform Your Mind

The chaos of daily life often sweeps us away from our center of calm. As you navigate the complexities of modern living, creating a sacred space dedicated to mindfulness can be your sanctuary. Establishing an environment that fosters peace and reflection isn't just beneficial—it's essential for maintaining mental clarity and emotional health. This chapter delves into the importance of designing such spaces, helping you cultivate areas that effectively support your mindfulness practices.

Creating a supportive environment is not about lavish decorations or expensive renovations; it's about simplicity and intentionality. A designated quiet zone, free from daily distractions, can significantly enhance your ability to focus and engage with mindfulness practices. Whether it's a small corner of your bedroom or a dedicated room, what matters is that the space feels safe and serene. Here, practicality meets purpose as you learn to transform any part of your home into a personal retreat that beckons you to pause and reconnect with yourself.

Establishing a personal sanctuary goes beyond physical space— creating an atmosphere that resonates with tranquility and inspiration. Soft lighting, comfortable seating, and personal items that evoke serenity (photos, inspirational quotes, or natural elements like plants or water) can enhance the ambiance. This chapter provides actionable advice on selecting elements that uplift and motivate you, ensuring your space reflects your needs and aesthetic preferences.

Moreover, the benefits of mindfulness aren't limited to solitary practice; they expand significantly when shared in a community. Exploring communal practice spaces, whether by joining existing groups or forming new ones, can offer profound connections with others on similar journeys. Sharing experiences and techniques enriches your practice and helps build a supportive network that fosters collective growth and learning.

Take control of your environment and how it influences your

mental state. Simple changes in your surroundings can profoundly impact your ability to manage stress and maintain mental focus. You can craft spaces and experiences that facilitate more profound mindfulness practices by actively engaging with this process.

This chapter is designed to guide and inspire you to take these steps toward creating your sacred spaces. It underscores the attainable nature of these practices within the confines of busy schedules and limited spaces. With each section geared towards actionable insights, you can start making effective changes immediately.

Embrace these strategies as tools for transformation—extensions of your commitment to living a more centered and mindful life. By understanding the importance of your surroundings in shaping your mental health, you harness the power to create lasting change—one space at a time.

Creating a supportive environment for mindfulness practice is essential for nurturing a consistent and effective routine. The spaces we inhabit have a profound impact on our mental well-being. Whether it's a corner of your bedroom, a cozy nook in the living room, or a dedicated room for meditation, crafting a space that encourages mindfulness can significantly enhance your practice. Consider lighting, decor, and minimal distractions to create an atmosphere conducive to inner reflection and peace.

Lighting plays a crucial role in setting the tone for your mindfulness practice. Natural light is ideal, fostering a sense of connection to the external world while promoting alertness. If natural light is limited, opt for soft, warm artificial lighting to create a calming ambiance. Dimmer switches or candles can also help adjust the light intensity to suit your mood. Experiment with different lighting options until you find what works best for you.

Incorporating elements of nature into your space can evoke feelings of tranquility and grounding. Consider adding plants, natural materials like wood or stone, or nature-inspired artwork to bring the outdoors inside. These elements can help foster a sense of calm and connectedness with the natural world, enhancing the overall mindfulness experience.

Minimizing distractions is critical to creating a space that supports deep focus and presence. Clear clutter, organize your surroundings, and remove any items that may distract your attention from the present moment. A clutter-free environment can promote mental clarity and reduce overwhelming feelings, allowing you to immerse yourself fully in your mindfulness practice.

Cultivating a Mindful Sanctuary

By consciously curating your space to align with your practice goals, you can enhance the quality of your meditation sessions and create a sanctuary for inner peace and reflection.

Creating a personal sanctuary conducive to meditation and reflection is a powerful way to enhance your mindfulness practice. Designating a specific area in your home or outdoors can help signal to your mind that it's time for introspection and mindfulness. This space should be free from distractions and clutter, allowing you to focus solely on your practice. Consider adding elements that promote relaxation, such as cushions, candles, or soothing artwork. These items can create a calming atmosphere supporting your inner peace journey.

Lighting plays a crucial role in setting the mood for mindfulness. Natural light is ideal but opt for soft, warm lighting instead of harsh overhead lights if it is impossible. Dimmer switches or lamps with adjustable brightness can help you customize the ambiance to suit your needs. Soft music or natural sounds can enhance the atmosphere and drown out background noise.

Incorporating elements of nature into your sanctuary can deepen your connection to the present moment. Plants, flowers, or even a small indoor fountain can bring a sense of tranquility and vitality to the space. Sitting near a window with a view of nature can also be incredibly grounding and rejuvenating.

Establishing a routine in your sanctuary can reinforce your commitment to mindfulness. Set aside dedicated time each day for meditation or reflection, even if it's just for a few minutes. Consistency is critical in developing a sustainable mindfulness practice, and creating a ritual around your practice signals to your brain that this time is sacred and non-negotiable.

Keep your sanctuary clean and organized to maintain a sense of peace and clarity. Clutter can distract and disrupt your focus, so make an effort to declutter regularly. Please spend some time tidying up your space daily, ensuring it remains a tranquil haven for introspection.

Remember that your sanctuary reflects your inner state, so treat it carefully and respectfully. By cultivating a nurturing environment for mindfulness, you are investing in your well-being and emotional balance. Allow yourself the gift of this sacred space to cultivate presence, peace, and self-awareness.

Descriptive Framework: Personal Mindfulness Environment

The Descriptive Framework for creating a personal mindfulness environment is a structured approach that assists individuals in designing and utilizing spaces conducive to mindfulness practices. It begins with identifying personal needs and preferences in a mindfulness space, considering sensory inputs like sound, sight, and smell. This initial step is crucial as it sets the foundation for a space that resonates with the individual's inner peace and tranquility.

Next, the framework guides individuals on physically setting up the space by selecting a specific room or corner dedicated to mindfulness practice. This involves minimizing clutter and choosing objects that evoke serenity, such as plants, stones, or simple art pieces. The physical arrangement significantly creates an atmosphere that promotes relaxation and focus during meditation or reflection sessions.

Once the space is established, the framework outlines incorporating this physical environment into mindfulness practice. It suggests routines to begin and end sessions effectively, helping individuals transition into a state of mindfulness seamlessly. By integrating the physical space with mindful activities, practitioners can enhance their overall experience and deepen their connection to the present moment.

Moreover, the framework emphasizes maintaining the sanctity of the space against daily disruptions. This involves setting boundaries to protect the space from external influences that may hinder mindfulness practice. Individuals can cultivate inner peace and balance amidst life's challenges by creating a haven for introspection and self-care.

Lastly, the framework encourages an iterative process of personal space refinement, prompting individuals to adapt to their environment as their mindfulness journey evolves. This flexibility allows continuous improvement and customization based on changing needs and preferences. By regularly revisiting and refining their mindfulness space, practitioners can ensure it remains a supportive sanctuary for mental well-being.

In summary, the Descriptive Framework for creating a personal mindfulness environment offers a structured approach to designing spaces that nurture mindfulness practices. Individuals can cultivate an environment that supports their journey towards inner peace and self-awareness by focusing on personal needs, physical setup, integration with practice routines, maintenance against disruptions, and iterative refinement.

Creating sacred spaces for mindfulness is not just about enhancing your immediate environment; it's about nurturing your mental and emotional well-being. By designing a supportive environment, you actively contribute to the quality of your mindfulness practice. A well-thought-out space can significantly diminish distractions and foster more profound, focused meditation.

Establishing a personal sanctuary goes beyond physical space—creating a refuge for your mind. This personal haven should resonate with peace and tranquility, enabling you to retreat from the day's stresses and reconnect with your inner self. It's essential for anyone looking to maintain balance in the hustle of daily life.

Moreover, the benefits of communal mindfulness practices cannot be overstated. Joining or forming a group provides a sense of community and support that can be incredibly empowering. Shared experiences in mindfulness practice help reinforce personal commitment and provide diverse perspectives that enrich your understanding and appreciation of mindfulness.

Take action today: start by identifying a small area in your home where you can be undisturbed, then personalize this space with items that evoke serenity and focus for you. Whether it's a favorite cushion, calming scents, or soothing sounds, make this space uniquely yours. Additionally, reach out to local or online communities dedicated to mindfulness; these can be invaluable resources as you forge your path toward greater peace and centeredness.

Remember, the journey to creating sacred spaces around and within you is ongoing. Embrace this process with patience and persistence. The rewards—enhanced clarity, increased calm, and heightened awareness—are worth the effort. Equip yourself with these mindful practices, and watch as they transform stress into serenity, not just in meditation but across all facets of life.

Chapter 13: Surmounting the Hurdles of Practice

"Mindfulness is a way of befriending

ourselves and our experience."

Jon Kabat-Zinn

When Daily Life Threatens Your Peace

Mindfulness practice is often envisioned as a serene endeavor, easily integrated into daily routines. However, the reality for many, especially busy women juggling multiple roles, is that maintaining such practices can feel like navigating a maze of obstacles. Understanding and overcoming these challenges is crucial to reaping the profound benefits of mindfulness.

The first significant obstacle many encounter is finding consistent time amidst a packed schedule. It's easy to prioritize immediate demands over the quiet pursuit of mindfulness. The key here is recognizing that even brief sessions can be profoundly beneficial. Initiating practice with just five minutes a day, perhaps at the start or end of your day, can create manageable yet impactful habits. The idea isn't to carve out large chunks of time initially but to build a foundation that naturally integrates into your life rhythms.

Another significant hurdle is maintaining motivation and commitment. Mindfulness might seem less urgent or feasible when stress peaks or personal crises occur. Here, it's essential to recall why you started practicing in the first place. Reflecting on moments when mindfulness has brought calm or clarity can reignite your motivation. Additionally, setting small, achievable goals can help maintain focus and provide a sense of accomplishment that fuels further practice.

Cultivating resilience in your approach to mindfulness means adapting your methods as circumstances change. A rigid practice schedule or technique might work one month but not the next. Being open to modifying your approach—whether trying different mindfulness exercises or shifting practice times—ensures that the practice remains relevant and supportive rather than another source of stress.

A practical strategy for sustaining mindfulness involves routine integration. Tying mindfulness practices to daily activities such as drinking morning coffee or commuting allows for regularity without overwhelming your schedule. This method also anchors mindfulness in everyday life, making it more tangible and accessible.

Engaging with a community or finding a mindfulness partner is also beneficial. Sharing experiences and challenges with others can provide new insights and reinforce commitment through mutual encouragement and accountability.

Lastly, leveraging technology can also aid consistency in practice. Numerous apps offer guided meditations, reminders, and tracking tools that help keep mindfulness at the forefront of daily activities—even amidst chaos.

By understanding these common obstacles and employing practical strategies to overcome them, you empower yourself to sustain a transformative practice that enhances calmness and resilience in chaotic moments. Remember, every small step is part of a more significant journey towards more profound peace and fulfillment.

Consistency in mindfulness practice can be challenging, especially when faced with the busyness of everyday life. Common obstacles such as lack of time, distractions, and wavering motivation can hinder one's commitment to regular mindfulness routines. Recognizing these hurdles and developing strategies to overcome them effectively is essential.

One obstacle many individuals face is finding the time to practice mindfulness amidst their hectic schedules. To overcome this challenge, it's crucial to prioritize mindfulness as a non-negotiable part of your day. Setting aside a few minutes in the morning or before bed can significantly improve your overall well-being. By viewing mindfulness practice as essential self-care, you can shift your mindset and make time for it, just like any other important task on your agenda.

Distractions are another common barrier to consistent mindfulness practice. Focusing on the present moment can be particularly challenging in today's fast-paced world of technology and constant stimuli. Creating a designated space for mindfulness practice free from distractions can help cultivate a sense of tranquility. Turning off notifications, finding a quiet corner, or using noise-canceling headphones can aid in maintaining focus during meditation or mindful activities.

Motivation is critical to sustaining a mindfulness practice over the long term. However, it's normal to experience fluctuations in motivation levels, especially during stressful or overwhelming periods. Reminding yourself of the benefits of mindfulness, such as reduced stress and increased emotional resilience, can reignite your commitment. Setting small, achievable goals and tracking progress can help maintain motivation and keep you accountable.

Incorporating mindfulness into daily routines may seem daunting initially, but perseverance and dedication can become a natural and rewarding habit. By acknowledging the common obstacles to consistent practice and implementing practical strategies to overcome them, you can surmount these hurdles and reap the numerous benefits of mindfulness.

Nurturing Motivation and Commitment in Mindfulness

Maintaining motivation and commitment to mindfulness practices can be challenging, especially when life presents its inevitable ups and downs. During these tumultuous times, our dedication to mindfulness is truly tested. Life's unpredictability may disrupt our routines, making it harder to find the time or energy to engage in mindfulness practices. However, mindfulness can offer the most significant benefits during these chaotic moments.

To stay motivated and committed, we must remind ourselves why we started this journey towards mindfulness in the first place. Reflect on the positive changes you have experienced since incorporating mindfulness. Acknowledge the moments of calm, clarity, and peace mindfulness has brought you amidst life's challenges.

Incorporating mindfulness into your daily routine can help solidify your commitment. Set aside specific times each day for your practice, whether in the morning before starting your day or in the evening before bed. Consistency is critical to reaping the full benefits of mindfulness.

During turbulent times, when stress levels are high, it can be tempting to push mindfulness practices aside. However, these are the moments when mindfulness can be most beneficial. Use mindfulness as a tool to navigate through difficult emotions and situations with grace and resilience. Rather than avoiding discomfort, face it head-on with a mindful attitude.

Surround yourself with a supportive community of like-minded individuals who can provide encouragement and accountability. Joining a meditation group or participating in online forums can help you stay motivated on your mindfulness journey. Sharing experiences and insights can deepen your practice and inspire continued commitment.

Practice self-compassion during challenging times when maintaining motivation feels particularly tough. Be gentle with yourself and recognize that setbacks are a natural part of any journey. Celebrate small victories along the way, acknowledging your progress, no matter how minor.

Remind yourself that your well-being is worth prioritizing. By investing time and effort into maintaining your mindfulness practice, you are investing in your mental and emotional health. Embrace the journey towards greater self-awareness and inner peace, knowing that each moment of practice brings you closer to a more centered and resilient way of being.

Stay committed, stay motivated, and remember that every moment of mindfulness brings you closer to a calmer, more centered existence.

In sustaining mindfulness practices, it is crucial to cultivate resilience and adaptability. Life is unpredictable, and challenges will inevitably arise, testing our commitment to mindfulness. However, we can navigate these obstacles gracefully by adopting a flexible mindset and resilient approach. Here are some practical strategies to help you stay grounded in your mindfulness journey amidst life's fluctuations.

1. Embrace Imperfection: Understand that consistency, not perfection, is critical in mindfulness practices. Allow yourself to miss a session or have a less focused practice. It's normal to have off days; what matters most is your commitment to returning to your practice without self-judgment.

2. Adapt Your Practice: Explore different mindfulness techniques and find what resonates with you. If sitting meditation feels challenging on a particular day, try mindful walking or deep breathing exercises instead. Flexibility in your practice ensures that you can maintain it even during hectic times.

3. Set Realistic Goals: Avoid overwhelming yourself with unrealistic expectations. Start small and gradually increase the duration or intensity of your practice as you build consistency. Celebrate small victories along the way, reinforcing your commitment to mindfulness.

4. Cultivate Self-Compassion: Be kind to yourself during setbacks or periods of inconsistency. Acknowledge any negative self-talk and replace it with words of encouragement. Remember that mindfulness is a journey, and self-compassion is essential.

5. Create a Supportive Environment: Surround yourself with like-minded individuals who value mindfulness. Join a

meditation group, attend workshops, or participate in online communities dedicated to mindfulness practices. Having a support system can help you stay motivated and accountable.

6. Reflect on Your Progress: Regularly reflect on how mindfulness has positively impacted your life. Notice any changes in your stress levels, emotional regulation, or overall well-being. These reflections can reinforce your dedication to continued practice.

7. Stay Open-Minded: Remain open to learning and growing in your mindfulness journey. Be willing to explore new techniques, perspectives, and insights that deepen your practice. An open mind fosters adaptability and resilience in the face of challenges.

By cultivating resilience and adaptability in your mindfulness practice, you equip yourself with the tools to navigate life's ups and downs more easily. Remember that consistency is vital, but flexibility is equally important in sustaining a fulfilling mindfulness journey over the long term.

As we wrap up this chapter, it's clear that the path to maintaining a consistent mindfulness practice is fraught with challenges. However, the strategies discussed here are designed to empower you, helping you navigate common obstacles with resilience and adaptability.

Firstly, recognizing and overcoming obstacles is crucial. Understanding these barriers is the first step towards mitigating them, whether it's lack of time, distractions, or waning interest. Implement simple tactics like scheduling short mindfulness sessions into your daily routine or creating a dedicated space for practice. These small changes can significantly impact your ability to stay consistent.

Secondly, keeping your motivation and commitment strong despite life's inevitable ups and downs is critical. Remember why you started practicing mindfulness in the first place. Perhaps it was to reduce stress, manage anxiety, or enjoy greater peace and presence. Revisit these reasons when your motivation dips. Additionally, tracking your progress or joining a mindfulness group can provide the encouragement needed to stay on track.

Lastly, the ability to cultivate resilience and adaptability in your practice ensures its sustainability. Mindfulness is not a one-size-fits-all solution; it requires tuning and adjustments as your life evolves. Be open to experimenting with different mindfulness exercises—meditation, mindful walking, or journaling—to find what resonates with you at other times.

Embrace these practices with patience and self-compassion. Remember, each small step is a more significant journey towards a more centered and joyful life. By actively engaging with these strategies, you are enhancing your well-being and setting a foundation for sustained peace and resilience in the face of chaos.

Keep moving forward with confidence in your ability to master these techniques. Each moment of mindfulness adds up, building towards a more serene and fulfilling life.

Chapter 14: The Mindful Path Forward

"To understand the immeasurable, the mind

must be extraordinarily quiet, still."

Jiddu Krishnamurti

The Future is Mindful: Embracing a Life of Intention and Harmony

As we navigate the final chapter of our journey towards mastering mindfulness amid life's relentless whirlwind, envisaging a future shaped by the principles and practices we've embraced becomes crucial. This chapter is not just a conclusion but a commencement—a portal to a life where mindfulness transcends being a mere practice to become the core of our existence. Here, we focus on setting goals for continuous growth, integrating mindfulness into our values, and envisioning a future where balanced, peaceful, and joyful mindfulness informs every aspect of life.

Setting goals is fundamental. It's about projecting your future self and shaping the pathway to get there. These aren't just any goals; they are reflections of a deeper understanding of who you are and who you aspire to be. This mindful approach to goal-setting transforms aspirations into tangible realities. It's about aligning your ambitions with your inner values, ensuring that each step forward is purposeful and enriching.

Integrating mindfulness into your lifestyle goes beyond occasional meditation or mindful breathing breaks during stressful times. It's about weaving this awareness through the fabric of your daily life—choosing relationships that foster positivity, adopting habits that nurture body and mind, and making career choices that resonate with your deepest values. Each decision is an opportunity to reinforce your commitment to a mindful way of living.

Envisioning a future dominated by mindfulness allows you to see potential challenges through a lens of composure and resilience. It involves anticipating how you might react to stressors and planning ways to engage with them mindfully. Imagine handling conflicts at work with calm assertiveness or embracing parenting challenges with patience and presence. This vision becomes a guiding star, keeping you aligned with your path no matter the obstacles.

The seamless integration of mindfulness throughout your life enhances personal peace and contributes significantly to the well-being of those around you. Your journey could inspire others, creating ripples that extend the benefits of mindfulness far beyond individual gains.

This chapter ties together all we have learned, reinforcing that the true essence of mindfulness is not found in solitary moments of meditation but in inconsistent application throughout every moment of our lives. The strategies discussed here are practical, designed for real-life application, and meant to empower you— transforming stress into serenity with every breath you take.

As we close this chapter, remember that each day offers new opportunities for practice and growth. The path forward is clear; it promises peace and fulfillment in every step taken mindfully. Embrace it wholeheartedly as you continue cultivating resilience, joy, and an unshakeable peace within the chaos that once seemed impossible.

As you continue your journey towards mindfulness and personal transformation, setting clear goals to guide your path forward is essential. Setting goals provides direction, motivation, and a sense of accomplishment as you progress in your practice. Begin by reflecting on where you are currently in your mindfulness journey and where you envision yourself in the future. Consider the areas of your life that could benefit from more mindfulness, whether managing stress, improving relationships, or enhancing overall well-being.

Set specific, measurable, achievable, relevant, and time-bound (SMART) goals to ensure your objectives are clear and attainable. For example, you might aim to meditate for 10 minutes daily, practice mindful breathing during stressful moments, or engage in a mindfulness course or workshop to deepen your understanding. You can make incremental progress and celebrate each achievement by breaking your goals into smaller steps.

Staying flexible and adapting your goals as needed is crucial, as well as recognizing that growth is a continuous process that may require adjustments over time. Be gentle with yourself if you encounter challenges or setbacks, and approach each moment with self-compassion and understanding. Remember that mindfulness is not about perfection but cultivating awareness and acceptance in the present moment.

As you set your sights on continued growth in mindfulness and personal transformation, envision the person you aspire to become, embodying qualities such as resilience, compassion, and inner peace. Allow these intentions to guide your daily actions and choices, aligning them with your values and deepest desires for a more fulfilling life. By setting meaningful goals, you empower yourself to take charge of your well-being and create a balanced, peaceful, and joy-filled future.

Weaving Mindfulness into Daily Life

Integrating mindfulness into your values and lifestyle choices is a transformative process that can lead to profound shifts in how you engage with the world around you. By weaving mindfulness into the fabric of your daily life, you create a foundation for greater peace, clarity, and resilience. Begin by setting intentions for how you want mindfulness to manifest. Whether through daily meditation, mindful eating, or intentional breathing exercises, consistency is vital in solidifying these practices as part of your routine.

Reflect on your core values and consider how mindfulness can support and enhance them. When you align your actions with your values, you cultivate a sense of authenticity and purpose in everything you do. Mindful decision-making becomes a natural extension of this alignment, allowing you to approach challenges with clarity and integrity.

Practice self-compassion as you navigate this journey of integration. Be gentle with yourself when setbacks occur, and remember that mindfulness is a lifelong practice filled with ups and downs. Embrace imperfection as an opportunity for growth rather than a failure, and allow yourself the space to learn and evolve.

As you incorporate mindfulness into your lifestyle choices, consider how it can positively impact your relationships, work environment, and overall well-being. Set boundaries to protect your mental and emotional energy, recognizing that self-care is not selfish but essential for sustainable growth. Create space for stillness amidst the noise of daily life, allowing yourself moments of quiet reflection to recharge and reconnect with your inner wisdom.

Integrate mindfulness into everyday activities like walking, cooking, or even driving. By bringing awareness to these moments, you infuse them with meaning and presence, cultivating a more profound sense of gratitude for the simple joys in life. Notice the beauty in the ordinary, finding moments of peace and joy amid chaos.

As mindfulness becomes woven into the tapestry of your existence, you may find that old patterns shift, relationships deepen, and clarity emerges where there was once confusion. Embrace this journey of transformation, knowing that each step taken mindfully brings you closer to a life filled with balance, peace, and joy. Allow yourself to surrender to the flow of change, trust in the process, and remain open to the endless possibilities that unfold when you live from a place of mindful awareness.

Envision a future where mindfulness informs all aspects of living, fostering a life of balance, peace, and joy. As you continue your mindful path forward, fully integrating mindfulness into your values and lifestyle choices is essential. This integration will create a harmonious relationship between your inner self and the external world, leading to a profound sense of alignment and purpose.

Set goals for continued growth in mindfulness and personal transformation. Consider what aspects of your life could benefit from a more mindful approach. Whether managing stress at work, improving relationships with loved ones, or simply finding peace in your daily routine, setting specific goals will help you stay focused and motivated. By consciously defining what you wish to achieve through mindfulness, you pave the way for meaningful change and growth.

Integrating mindfulness into personal values and lifestyle choices involves making conscious decisions that align with your newfound awareness. This may mean choosing activities that nourish your mind, body, and spirit or setting boundaries that prioritize your well-being. By weaving mindfulness into the fabric of your daily life, you create a solid foundation for lasting transformation.

Envisioning a future where mindfulness informs all aspects of living is about painting a vivid picture of the life you desire. Imagine responding to challenges calmly and clearly, embracing each moment with presence and gratitude. Visualize a future where balance, peace, and joy are not just fleeting moments but integral parts of your existence, guiding you through calm and stormy waters.

As you move forward on this mindful path, remember that transformation is a continual process. By setting clear intentions, integrating mindfulness into your values, and envisioning a future guided by balance and joy, you empower yourself to create the life you desire. Embrace each step with openness and curiosity, knowing that every moment holds the potential for growth and enlightenment.

As we close to the end of our journey, let's reflect on what we've explored and how it can profoundly shape your life. Mindfulness is a practice and a transformational path that intertwines deeply with your values and everyday choices. It offers you a powerful tool to navigate through life's turbulence with grace and composure, fostering peace that permeates all aspects of your existence.

Embracing mindfulness entirely means making it a core part of your daily living, allowing it to guide your decisions and interactions. This commitment to incorporating mindfulness into your life is crucial. It ensures that the serenity and joy you cultivate in your quiet moments are also present in the bustling activity of your daily routines. You continually nurture and expand this enriching practice by setting clear goals for ongoing growth.

Visualize a future where mindfulness is your constant companion, shaping how you perceive and interact with the world. Imagine facing challenges not with trepidation but with a poised readiness. Each moment is met with a balanced response in this envisioned future, contributing to a life experience characterized by deep fulfillment and happiness.

The strategies we've discussed are designed not only for immediate relief but also for sustainable growth. They are practical, straightforward, and tailored to fit even the busiest schedules. Implementing these practices empowers you to reclaim control over your mental and emotional landscape, transforming stress into serenity.

Remember, the journey towards mindfulness is uniquely yours, but know that you are not alone in this pursuit. Countless others are on similar paths, seeking to find calm in the chaos of their lives. Stay committed to your practice, be patient, and continually seek ways to integrate these lessons into every facet of your life.

Let each step forward on this path be taken with intention and confidence, knowing that each moment of mindfulness significantly transforms how you live and enjoy your life. Here's to moving forward with awareness, purpose, and joy.

Epilogue

"Only in the oasis of silence can we drink deeply

from our inner cup of wisdom."

Sue Patton Thoele

Embracing Serenity: A Journey Towards Joyful Living

As we conclude our journey together, we must reflect on the transformative path we've embarked upon. You've been equipped with a treasure trove of mindfulness techniques and strategies designed to help you navigate the stormy seas of daily life with grace and resilience. Remember, the essence of mindfulness is not in eradicating life's chaos but transforming your reaction to it.

Incorporating the principles discussed can significantly enhance your quality of life. By applying these mindful practices, you can expect to see a reduction in stress, an increase in your overall emotional well-being, and a newfound joy in life's simple moments. Whether through mindful breathing during a hectic day or practicing gratitude before bed, each small step is a leap towards a more serene and joyful existence.

We revisited several critical concepts throughout this book: the power of presence, the art of acceptance, and the strength of stillness. These are not just ideas but practical tools that you can wield to craft a more peaceful life amid everyday chaos.

Consider integrating these practices into your daily routine to benefit from this book. Start small—perhaps with five minutes of meditation each day—and gradually increase as you become more comfortable. Use mindfulness as a lens through which you view your challenges and moments of joy and connection.

It's important to acknowledge that this journey isn't free from obstacles. Mindfulness is a skill that requires patience and persistence to develop. Some days will be easier than others, and that's perfectly okay. The goal isn't perfection; it's progress.

Taking Mindful Steps Forward

As you continue to apply these insights, remember that every moment offers a new opportunity for practice. Whether dealing with work stress, family dynamics, or personal challenges, mindfulness provides a place to operate calmly.

Encourage yourself to keep exploring this path even after turning the last page of this book. There is always more to learn about oneself and new depths of peace. If you find yourself struggling or if certain aspects of mindfulness seem elusive, consider seeking out communities or experts who can offer guidance and support.

In closing, let me remind you that your ability to navigate life's complexities with mindfulness is about enhancing personal happiness and contributing positively to the lives around you. As you cultivate serenity within, it radiates outward, influencing all facets of your life—from personal relationships to professional endeavors.

Remember, every breath is an opportunity to reset and reconnect with your center. Trust in your power to transform stress into serenity and reclaim joy in your life.

"The mind is everything. What you think you become."

Buddha

This quote encapsulates our discussions beautifully: by fostering mindfulness, you shape your perceptions and the reality around you. Here's to finding calm in the chaos and transforming each moment into an opportunity for growth and joy.

Conclusion

"The real meditation is how you live your life."

Jon Kabat-Zinn

In conclusion, exploring mindfulness within these pages extends beyond a simple practice; it represents a shift towards a more conscious and deliberate way of living. This book not only introduces readers to the principles of mindfulness but also guides them through the practical application of these principles in daily life. By demystifying mindfulness and making it accessible, we have laid a foundation for anyone willing to engage in this transformative practice.

- As we've seen, mindfulness is not a destination but a continuous journey that enriches our lives in myriad ways. By fostering an awareness of the present moment, we open ourselves to life's fullness, embracing its challenges and joys.

- The practices detailed in this book serve as starting points for each individual to explore the unique contours of their mindfulness path. Whether through meditation, mindful breathing, or the art of acceptance, these techniques are tools to build a life of presence, compassion, and peace.

Beyond the individual, mindfulness can potentially alter the fabric of our communities and society. When we approach our interactions with others from a place of mindfulness, we contribute to a more compassionate, understanding, and tolerant world.

- Furthermore, the environmental implications of mindfulness remind us that our well-being is intimately connected with the health of our planet. By living more mindfully, we make choices that support sustainability and ecological balance, reflecting a deep respect for the interconnectedness of all life.

This conclusion invites readers to absorb the teachings within these pages and live them out daily. The true essence of mindfulness reveals itself in the day-to-day, moment-to-moment experiences. As we continue to practice, we will find that mindfulness becomes less of something we do and more of who we are.

- Finally, as we move forward, may we understand that each moment holds the potential for mindfulness. Each breath, step, and interaction is an opportunity to practice presence, cultivate inner peace, and contribute to the well-being of the world around us.

This book does not conclude in the spirit of mindfulness on its final page. Instead, it begins a personal and collective exploration into a more mindful existence. With each reader's journey, the ripple effects of mindfulness extend further, touching lives and transforming communities.

- Allow the insights and practices shared here to guide you toward greater awareness and serenity. Remember, the path of mindfulness is personal and unique to each individual's experience and circumstance.

With this, we close a chapter in a book and open the door to a new way of being that embraces mindfulness in all its depth and beauty. May your journey be filled with discovery, growth, and profound peace.

Bonus Material

Your Questions, Answered!

1. How Can I Apply Mindfulness Techniques in High-Stress Situations, Like Work Emergencies or Family Crises?

Applying mindfulness techniques in high-stress situations, such as work emergencies or family crises, may initially seem challenging. Yet, mindfulness can genuinely shine in these intense moments and offer its most profound benefits. The essence of mindfulness—being present and fully engaging with the here and now, without judgment—can be a powerful tool in navigating stressful situations with more calmness and clarity.

When faced with an emergent situation at work or a family crisis, the first step is to ground yourself using mindful breathing. This process involves taking a few deep breaths to center your attention and calm the initial surge of stress or panic. By focusing on the rhythm of your breath, you create a brief pause that allows you to respond to the situation more thoughtfully rather than impulsively. This practice doesn't just help mitigate the physiological responses to stress, such as elevated heart rate and rapid breathing, but also promotes mental clarity, enabling you to assess the situation more objectively.

Beyond breath work, mindfulness encourages cultivating an observer's perspective, where you acknowledge your thoughts and emotions without becoming overwhelmed. This can be particularly useful in a highly stressful situation. By recognizing your emotional responses without judgment, you can prevent them from dictating your actions, for example, acknowledging feelings of frustration or anxiety but focusing on solving the problem rather than the emotions themselves. Similarly, mindfulness can enhance communication during a crisis by fostering a more compassionate and empathetic approach towards yourself and others involved.

Incorporating mindfulness techniques in such scenarios also involves a practice of acceptance. Acceptance in this context doesn't mean resigning to the situation but facing it with an open mind, without resistance or denial. This approach can reduce the additional stress from wishing things were different or ruminating on what should have been done. Instead, acceptance allows you to engage with the situation as it is, often making it easier to identify practical steps to address the challenge.

Applying mindfulness in high-stress situations is about maintaining a presence of mind despite the chaos. It involves harnessing the ability to remain focused, composed, and compassionate, allowing for more effective problem-solving and decision-making. Significantly, like any skill, the effectiveness of mindfulness under pressure improves with practice. Regular mindfulness practice, even in moments of calm, builds your resilience and equips you with the tools to tackle stressors more effectively when they arise.

2. What Are Some Common Misconceptions About Mindfulness That Beginners Should Be Aware Of?

One common misconception about mindfulness is the belief that it requires an individual to empty their mind of thoughts. This misunderstanding can lead beginners to become frustrated when they find themselves unable to achieve a prominent mind during meditation or mindfulness practices. However, the essence of mindfulness is not about eliminating thoughts but rather about observing them without attachment or judgment. It's about learning to be present with whatever arises in the mind, acknowledging thoughts as they come, and then letting them go quickly, turning the attention back to the present moment, such as the breath, bodily sensations, or the immediate environment.

Another misconception is that mindfulness practice is only suitable or effective when done in silence, seated on a cushion for lengthy periods. This belief may deter individuals with busy schedules or those who struggle with traditional seated meditation. Mindfulness, however, is a flexible practice that can be incorporated into daily life in various ways, not just during formal meditation. Simple activities like mindful walking, eating, or even engaging in routine tasks can become acts of mindfulness when done with intention and total awareness. This adaptability makes mindfulness accessible to everyone, regardless of lifestyle or preferences.

Finally, some beginners may mistakenly think that mindfulness is a quick fix for deep-seated psychological issues or stress. While mindfulness has been shown to reduce stress and improve mental health, it is not an instant solution to all life's problems. The benefits of mindfulness build over time with consistent practice and can significantly enhance one's quality of life, resilience, and well-being. However, expecting instantaneous results can lead to disillusionment and abandonment of the practice. Understanding that mindfulness is a skill that deepens and unfolds gradually helps set realistic expectations for beginners.

Addressing these misconceptions early on can assist those new to mindfulness, ensuring a more informed, patient, and compassionate approach to their practice. By recognizing that mindfulness is a journey rather than a destination, beginners can cultivate a more meaningful and sustainable practice, leading to a more profound sense of peace, awareness, and connection to the present moment.

3. Can Practicing Mindfulness Help With Chronic Pain or Illness, and if So, How?

Mindfulness has been increasingly recognized as a beneficial strategy in managing chronic pain and illness, offering a nonpharmacological approach that can significantly improve quality of life. The essence of mindfulness, being fully present and engaged in the current moment without judgment, allows individuals suffering from chronic conditions to alter their relationship with pain and discomfort. Rather than focusing on the elimination of pain, which is often the primary approach in conventional treatment models, mindfulness encourages a compassionate and observant stance toward one's experiences of pain. This shift in perception can lead to a decrease in the intensity of pain experienced and enhance one's ability to cope with ongoing discomfort.

The mechanism behind mindfulness' effectiveness in pain management is multifaceted. Firstly, mindfulness practice, including meditation, can lead to changes in the brain regions associated with pain perception, notably reducing activity in areas linked to pain's cognitive and emotional aspects. This means that while the physical sensation may remain, its distressing impact is lessened, allowing individuals to experience pain less overwhelmingly. Additionally, mindfulness fosters a reduction in stress and anxiety, which are often exacerbated by chronic pain and can contribute to a vicious cycle of increased pain sensations and emotional distress. By mitigating these reactions, mindfulness can break this cycle, leading to improved emotional well-being and potentially reducing the subjective experience of pain.

Furthermore, mindfulness teaches individuals to distinguish between the primary sensation of pain and the secondary reactions, such as the emotional and cognitive responses that often amplify suffering. By recognizing and gently disengaging from these reactive patterns, individuals can reduce the layers of suffering added to the raw pain sensation. Regular mindfulness practice can also enhance one's resilience and ability to engage in daily activities despite chronic conditions, fostering a sense of empowerment and reducing feelings of helplessness that often accompany long-term illness.

In conclusion, while mindfulness may not cure chronic pain or illness, it offers powerful tools for managing these conditions more effectively. By changing how individuals relate to pain, reducing stress, and increasing resilience, mindfulness can improve quality of life, even in the face of ongoing health challenges. It's crucial for those exploring mindfulness for pain management to approach the practice with patience and without the expectation of immediate relief, as the benefits of mindfulness build gradually and are most profound with consistent practice over time.

4. Is There a Way to Integrate Mindfulness Practices for Children, and What Benefits Might They Experience?

Integrating mindfulness practices for children can be profoundly beneficial, offering them tools to manage stress, enhance focus, and cultivate emotional resilience from an early age. The process involves teaching children simple mindfulness exercises tailored to their developmental level, such as mindful breathing, listening, eating, and walking. These activities encourage children to pay attention to the present moment non-judgmentally, noticing their thoughts, feelings, and bodily sensations as they occur. By learning to observe their experiences with curiosity rather than react automatically, children can develop a greater sense of self-awareness and control over their responses to the world around them.

One of the key benefits of mindfulness for children is improved emotional regulation. Through mindfulness exercises, children learn to recognize and name their emotions, understanding that feelings are transient and that they can manage them constructively. This ability to 'pause' before reacting can help reduce impulsivity, tantrums, and aggression, leading to better relationships with peers and adults. Furthermore, mindfulness practices have been shown to enhance focus and attention in children, making it easier for them to concentrate on tasks and engage in learning. This can be particularly beneficial in educational settings, where distractions are frequent, and the ability to stay focused is linked to academic success.

Additionally, mindfulness can be crucial in reducing stress and anxiety in children. In a world where children are increasingly exposed to stimuli and pressures from school and social media, mindfulness can calm the mind and body. Techniques such as mindful breathing can provide children with a practical tool to cope with stress, fostering a sense of inner peace and resilience that can support their mental well-being throughout their lives. Furthermore, by incorporating mindfulness into daily routines, children can cultivate a greater appreciation for life's simple pleasures, enhancing their overall happiness and well-being.

Incorporating mindfulness into the lives of children requires commitment and creativity, often involving the participation of parents, educators, and caregivers. However, the effort to integrate these practices at a young age can lay the foundation for a lifetime of mindfulness benefits, equipping children with the skills to navigate the complexities of life with calmness, empathy, and awareness.

5. How Might Someone Who is Skeptical About Mindfulness Be Convinced of Its Benefits?

To address skepticism towards mindfulness, it's practical to present scientific evidence and personal testimonies highlighting the tangible benefits of mindfulness practices. The growing body of research supports mindfulness as a beneficial tool for mental health, showing measurable changes in brain regions associated with attention, emotion regulation, and stress response. For instance, neuroimaging studies have demonstrated that regular mindfulness meditation can increase density in the prefrontal cortex, an area of the brain linked to higher-order brain functions such as awareness, concentration, and decision-making. This evidence provides a biological basis for many individuals' cognitive improvements after practicing mindfulness.

In addition to scientific evidence, sharing personal stories and testimonials can be particularly compelling. Hearing how individuals have transformed their approach to stress, anxiety, and overall emotional well-being through mindfulness can resonate on a personal level. These narratives often highlight the practical benefits of mindfulness in everyday life, such as improved relationships, enhanced focus, and greater emotional resilience. Skeptics may find it easier to relate to personal experiences and real-life examples of how mindfulness has been beneficial, making the concept more accessible and appealing.

For those skeptical about the abstract aspects of mindfulness, emphasizing its practical applications can be effective. Mindfulness can be integrated into daily activities without special equipment or significant time commitments, making it a versatile tool for stress management and self-improvement. Practices such as mindful eating, walking, or even breathing exercises during a busy day can serve as entry points for skeptics to experience mindfulness in a non-threatening, straightforward manner. By starting with these simple practices, individuals may notice subtle improvements in their well-being, motivating further exploration and deeper engagement with mindfulness techniques. This approach allows skeptics to verify mindfulness's benefits through personal experience, often the most convincing evidence of all.

6. What Are the Scientific Studies or Evidence Supporting the Effectiveness of Mindfulness?

Numerous scientific studies have provided a strong foundation of evidence supporting the effectiveness of mindfulness in enhancing mental health and cognitive functioning. One of the most compelling pieces of evidence comes from neuroimaging studies, which have observed physical changes in the brain's structure and function among individuals who practice mindfulness meditation regularly. For example, research has shown increased gray matter density in the hippocampus, known for its role in learning and memory and structures associated with self-awareness, compassion, and introspection. Additionally, decreases in gray matter density have been observed in the amygdala, which plays a significant role in anxiety and stress responses. These changes suggest mindfulness can enhance cognitive functions and emotional regulation by physically remodeling the brain.

Further supporting the effectiveness of mindfulness are studies focusing on its impact on psychological well-being and physical health. Research has indicated that mindfulness meditation can lead to significant reductions in symptoms of anxiety and depression, outcomes attributed to mindfulness's ability to enhance emotion regulation strategies and reduce rumination. Furthermore, mindfulness practices have been linked to improved physical health markers, including reduced blood pressure, improved immune response, and decreased chronic pain intensity. These improvements in psychological and physical health demonstrate mindfulness's broad applications and provide a robust argument for its effectiveness as a therapeutic intervention.

Beyond individual studies, systematic reviews and meta-analyses have aggregated data from multiple research projects, further validating the effectiveness of mindfulness. These comprehensive reviews have consistently found that mindfulness-based interventions can produce measurable improvements in a wide range of psychological conditions, including stress, depression, anxiety, and post-traumatic stress disorder (PTSD). By analyzing the cumulative evidence, these analyses offer robust and objective confirmation of the beneficial effects of mindfulness across different populations and settings. The growing body of scientific research not only underscores the significant positive impacts that mindfulness can have on mental and physical health but also reinforces its value as a practical tool for improving overall well-being and quality of life.

7. Does Mindfulness Practice Require a Specific Amount of Time Each Day to Be Beneficial?

The question of whether mindfulness practice necessitates a specific daily duration to yield benefits is significant, especially for individuals struggling to find time in their hectic schedules. Research indicates that the effectiveness of mindfulness does not necessarily correlate with long, drawn-out sessions of meditation or practice. Instead, even brief periods of mindfulness exercises can confer noticeable benefits to one's mental and physical health. Studies have demonstrated that as little as a few minutes per day can enhance focus, reduce stress levels, and improve emotional regulation. This flexibility makes mindfulness an accessible tool for many people, irrespective of their lifestyle or time constraints.

Mindfulness practices, such as focused breathing, mindfulness meditation, and mindful walking, can be versatilely integrated into daily routines. For instance, dedicating just a few minutes in the morning to mindfulness can set a positive tone for the day, fostering a sense of calm and presence that benefits mental clarity and emotional resilience. Similarly, brief mindfulness exercises during the day, like focusing entirely on the task at hand or engaging in a short meditation or deep-breathing session, can effectively manage stress and enhance productivity. This modular approach allows individuals to tailor their mindfulness practice to fit their unique schedule and needs, making it more likely for them to maintain the habit long-term.

In conclusion, the duration of daily mindfulness practice is less critical than the consistency and intention behind the practice. Regular engagement, even for short periods, can cumulate significant benefits over time, contributing to reduced stress, improved cognitive function, and better overall well-being. This flexibility in practice duration demystifies mindfulness for beginners and supports the idea that mindfulness is a highly adaptable, personal practice that can evolve with an individual's lifestyle and preferences. This adaptability ensures that mindfulness remains a practical and accessible tool for enhancing the quality of life in the modern world.

8. How Does One Handle the Challenge of Maintaining Regular Mindfulness Practice Amidst a Busy Schedule?

Maintaining a regular mindfulness practice amidst a busy schedule is a challenge many people face, but it's crucial for the consistent and effective incorporation of mindfulness into one's life. To meet this challenge, adopting a flexible and practical approach to mindfulness is essential, recognizing that the quality of mindfulness practice often outweighs the quantity. Incorporating mindfulness into daily activities can make the training more accessible and sustainable. This could mean taking short breaks throughout the day to focus on breathing, being fully present during routine activities like eating or walking or using mindfulness apps during commutes. Such integrated practices can ensure that mindfulness becomes a seamless part of one's day rather than feeling like an additional task on an already full agenda.

Additionally, setting realistic expectations and goals for mindfulness practice is vital to overcoming the challenge of a busy schedule. Rather than aiming for lengthy sessions that might be difficult to accommodate, individuals can start with short periods of mindfulness and gradually increase the duration as it becomes a more natural part of their routine. It's also beneficial to be kind to oneself when occasional lapses occur, understanding that consistency over time is more important than perfection in each session. Establishing a specific time and place for mindfulness practice can help create a habit, making it easier to maintain regularity. For instance, practicing mindfulness for a few minutes every morning before starting the day or in the evening to wind down can anchor the habit in daily life.

Finally, leveraging technology can also assist in maintaining a regular mindfulness practice. Numerous apps and online platforms offer guided mindfulness exercises that can be easily incorporated into one's daily schedule, regardless of how cramped. These resources can provide the structure and variety needed to stay engaged with the practice and make it easier to commit to regular sessions. Furthermore, mindfulness can be practiced in various settings, not just in quiet rooms but also in nature or the workplace during breaks. This adaptability means that individuals can find moments for mindfulness even amid a hectic day, turning the challenge of a busy schedule into an opportunity for regular, short mindfulness practices that contribute to well-being and stress management.

9. Can Mindfulness Improve Relationships, and What Practices Specifically Target Interpersonal Connections?

Mindfulness has been shown to significantly enhance the quality of interpersonal relationships by emphasizing present-moment awareness and non-judgmental acceptance. This impact is rooted in how mindfulness cultivates a deeper understanding of oneself and others, fostering a sense of empathy and connection crucial for healthy relationships. By practicing mindfulness, individuals can develop the ability to respond to situations calmly rather than reacting impulsively based on emotions. This can reduce conflicts and enhance communication by encouraging a more compassionate and empathetic interaction approach.

Specific mindfulness practices designed to improve relationships include mindful listening, expressing gratitude, and engaging in mindful conversation. Mindful listening involves fully concentrating on the speaker without formulating a response while still talking, demonstrating respect and care for the other person's thoughts and feelings. This can lead to more meaningful and less confrontational exchanges, as both parties feel heard and understood. Expressing gratitude mindfully involves consciously acknowledging the positive aspects of relationships and verbalizing appreciation for the other person, which can strengthen bonds and increase mutual respect.

Additionally, engaging in mindful conversations where each

person is fully present can significantly enhance the quality of interactions. This means putting aside distractions, making eye contact, and fully engaging in conversation. Such mindfulness practices improve communication and deepen the connection between individuals by fostering a shared sense of presence and attentiveness. Over time, these practices can lead to more satisfying and supportive relationships as both parties become more attuned to each other's needs and responsive in a constructive manner.

In summary, mindfulness can profoundly impact relationships by improving communication, increasing empathy, and fostering a deeper connection between individuals. Individuals can transform their relationships into more nurturing, understanding, and supportive engagements by integrating specific mindfulness practices into daily interactions. These benefits are not limited to personal relationships but can extend to professional and casual relationships, making mindfulness a valuable tool for enhancing interpersonal connections across all areas of life.

10. What Role Does Mindfulness Play in Overcoming Addiction or Self-Destructive Behaviors?

Mindfulness plays a pivotal role in overcoming addiction and self-destructive behaviors by fostering self-awareness and creating a space between thoughts and actions. This gap allows individuals to observe their cravings or impulses without immediate reaction, providing an opportunity to make more conscious choices. In the context of addiction, mindfulness helps individuals recognize the triggers and patterns of their behavior, understanding that cravings are temporary and that they can observe these feelings without needing to act on them. This awareness is crucial in breaking the cycle of addiction, as it empowers the person to respond to discomfort or emotional pain with healthier coping mechanisms rather than substance use or self-destructive behaviors.

Furthermore, mindfulness techniques teach individuals how to manage stress and negative emotions in a non-judgmental way, reducing the reliance on addictive behaviors as a form of escape. By practicing mindfulness, people can learn to tolerate difficult emotions and discomfort, gradually decreasing the intensity and impact of cravings. This is essential in the recovery process, as it addresses not only the physical aspect of addiction but also the emotional and psychological components. The practice of mindfulness encourages a kind and compassionate attitude towards oneself, which is especially important in overcoming the shame and guilt often associated with addiction. This self-compassion fosters a positive self-image and supports the recovery process.

In addition to the individual benefits, mindfulness can also enhance the effectiveness of other treatments for addiction. It is often combined with cognitive-behavioral therapy to amplify the treatment effects by increasing mental resilience and emotional regulation. Mindfulness-based relapse prevention programs have been developed to specifically target the challenges faced during recovery, teaching strategies to handle triggers and cravings effectively. Through regular practice, mindfulness strengthens the mind's ability to concentrate and stay present, which is beneficial in maintaining sobriety and preventing relapse.

Integrating mindfulness into the recovery process can lead to profound changes in how individuals perceive themselves and their ability to change their behaviors. It nurtures a more compassionate and understanding relationship with oneself and enhances the capacity to make life-affirming choices free from addiction and self-destruction. By building a solid foundation of mindfulness, individuals equip themselves with the necessary tools to navigate the complexities of recovery and foster a life of balance, well-being, and freedom from addictive behaviors.

11.   Are There Mindfulness Practices That Can Specifically Help With Anxiety and Depression?

Certainly, mindfulness practices can be particularly effective in managing and alleviating symptoms of anxiety and depression. These mental health conditions often arise from persistent patterns of negative thinking, excessive worry about the future, or rumination on the past. At its core, mindfulness encourages living in the present moment and observing thoughts and feelings without judgment. This can be remarkably liberating for those struggling with anxiety and depression, as it offers a way to break free from the cycle of negative thought patterns that fuel these conditions.

Mindfulness techniques such as meditation, mindful breathing, and body scans help individuals anchor their attention in the present, reducing the tendency to worry about future events or dwell on past incidents. For example, meditation guides the mind to focus on a single point of reference, such as the breath, which can help calm the mind and reduce stress. This practice can create a sense of inner peace and stability, offering a refuge from the turbulent emotions and thoughts associated with anxiety and depression. Mindful breathing, in particular, can be a quick and effective method for reducing immediate anxiety or panic by slowing down the heart rate and promoting relaxation.

Body scans further enhance mindfulness by encouraging individuals to become more attuned to their physical sensations in a non-judgmental manner. This can be especially helpful in identifying tension or discomfort in the body that may be associated with emotional distress. By gradually working through each part of the body, individuals can learn to release physical tension and, by extension, ease mental stress. The practice of mindfulness not only offers immediate relief from symptoms but also fosters long-term changes in how individuals relate to their thoughts and feelings. Over time, regular mindfulness practice can help develop a more compassionate and gentle approach towards oneself, reducing the impact of negative self-talk and boosting overall mental health.

In addition to these practices, incorporating mindfulness into daily activities can enhance the benefits further. Individuals can consciously bring attention to routine tasks—such as eating, walking, or even washing dishes—to cultivate mindfulness throughout the day. This ongoing practice helps to reinforce the habit of living in the present moment, making it easier to manage anxiety and depression. In essence, mindfulness offers a powerful and accessible tool for improving mental health, providing both immediate relief and long-term resilience against the challenges of anxiety and depression.

12.   How Can Mindfulness Be Adapted for People With Attention Disorders or Difficulty Focusing?

Mindfulness practices can be particularly beneficial for individuals with attention disorders, such as Attention Deficit Hyperactivity Disorder (ADHD), who may struggle with focusing, impulsivity, and maintaining attention on tasks at hand. The nature of mindfulness—focusing on the present moment with acceptance and without judgment—can provide a structured way for those with attention disorders to gradually learn how to enhance their focus and attention span.

Adapting mindfulness for those with difficulty focusing involves several key considerations. First, starting with shorter, more engaging mindfulness exercises that can easily hold their attention may be beneficial. For instance, mindful listening to music or brief guided meditations can be effective starting points that don't require long periods of stillness or silence, which might be challenging initially. These activities can be gentle introductions to directing and maintaining attention on a single focus point.

Further personalization of mindfulness practices can include using mindfulness apps designed specifically for individuals with ADHD or similar conditions. These apps often feature a variety of mindfulness exercises adapted to different needs and attention spans, offering visual or auditory cues to guide users gently back to the task when their mind wanders. In addition to using technology, incorporating physical movement into mindfulness practice, such as mindful walking or gentle yoga, can also be beneficial. These practices allow for the release of excess energy and make it easier for individuals with attention disorders to engage in mindfulness without feeling constrained by stillness.

Over time, with regular and consistent practice, mindfulness can help improve the ability to concentrate and reduce impulsiveness. It equips individuals with the tools to notice when their attention is drifting and to bring their focus back to the present moment non-judgmentally. This improved self-regulation and awareness can have profound effects not only on attention and focus but also on overall emotional and psychological well-being.

However, It is essential to approach mindfulness practice with patience and adjust expectations. Progress may be slow and non-linear, particularly for those with attention disorders. Celebrating small victories and incremental improvements can encourage persistence in the practice. By adapting mindfulness techniques to meet their unique needs and challenges, individuals with attention disorders can gain significant benefits, enhancing their ability to focus, manage stress, and live more fully in the present moment.

13. What Are the Differences Between Mindfulness and Other Forms of Meditation or Mental Health Practices?

Mindfulness, while often integrated into various meditation practices, distinguishes itself by its focus on the present moment and the cultivation of a non-judgmental awareness of one's thoughts, feelings, and bodily sensations. Unlike other meditation practices that might involve the repetition of a mantra, visualization, or pursuing a transcendent state, mindfulness emphasizes being fully present and engaged with whatever is happening in the here and now. This form of meditation does not attempt to change or manipulate the current state of mind but rather to observe it with kindness and curiosity. This approach helps individuals develop a deeper understanding of their mental patterns and enables them to respond more effectively to stress rather than reacting automatically based on ingrained habits.

Comparatively, other mental health practices, such as cognitive-behavioral therapy (CBT), also offer tools for managing stress and improving mental health but do so through structurally different approaches. CBT focuses on identifying and challenging distorted or negative thought patterns and behaviors and then applying strategies to change these patterns. While mindfulness may be incorporated as a component of CBT to enhance self-awareness, CBT is more directive and problem-solving, aiming to alter thought and behavior patterns causing emotional distress.

The effectiveness of mindfulness comes from its capacity to enhance moment-to-moment awareness, which can transform one's relationship with one's mental and emotional experiences. By fostering a stance of openness and curiosity towards whatever arises in consciousness, mindfulness encourages a shift from identifying with thoughts and feelings to recognizing them as passing events in the mind. This shift can lead to reduced emotional reactivity and an increased sense of calm and emotional resilience. On the other hand, other mental health practices, including different forms of meditation, might target specific outcomes, such as relaxation, enhanced concentration, or spiritual growth, offering diverse paths according to individual needs and preferences.

While mindfulness shares some commonalities with other forms of meditation and mental health practices, its distinct emphasis on present-moment awareness and non-judgment sets it apart. This unique approach helps individuals cultivate a different relationship with their internal experience, offering benefits complementary to those found in other mental health and meditative disciplines.

14.   How Can Mindfulness Impact Physical Health, Such as Blood Pressure or Immune Function?

The relationship between mindfulness and physical health, particularly concerning blood pressure and immune function, reveals a fascinating intersection between the mind and the body. Research suggests that regular mindfulness meditation can positively affect physical health, mainly by reducing stress levels closely linked with hypertension and compromised immune function. Stress activates the body's "fight or flight" response, leading to a cascade of physiological effects, including increased heart rate and blood pressure and a suppression of the immune system. Mindfulness practices help mitigate these stress responses, potentially lowering blood pressure and enhancing immune function.

Mindfulness encourages individuals to focus on the present moment in a non-judgmental manner. This focus can interrupt the chain of habitual stress reactions by fostering a relaxation response in the body. For example, guided mindfulness exercises often involve deep breathing techniques, which can directly influence the parasympathetic nervous system, decreasing heart rate and blood pressure. Over time, this relaxation can contribute to sustained improvements in cardiovascular health. Additionally, the stress-reduction benefits of mindfulness may contribute to improving immune function. Chronic stress can lead to inflammation and weaken the immune system, making the body more susceptible to infections and diseases. By reducing stress, mindfulness practices can help lower inflammation and enhance the body's immune response.

Furthermore, mindfulness can increase awareness of lifestyle habits contributing to high blood pressure and poor immune function, such as poor diet, lack of exercise, and inadequate sleep. By becoming more aware of these habits, individuals may be inspired to adopt healthier lifestyle choices, further supporting physical health. Also, several studies have demonstrated that mindfulness meditation can lead to changes in the brain and body that positively affect health markers. For instance, mindfulness practices have been associated with reduced levels of pro-inflammatory genes, which can contribute to a healthier immune system, and changes in brain areas related to stress regulation, emotion control, and self-awareness, which can indirectly influence physical well-being.

In summary, mindfulness offers a promising pathway for improving physical health by directly reducing stress responses that impact blood pressure and immune function and promoting healthier lifestyle choices through increased self-awareness. While further research is needed to understand the mechanisms behind these effects fully, current evidence supports the integration of mindfulness practices as a complementary approach to maintaining and enhancing physical health.

15.   Can Mindfulness Practice Lead to Tangible Changes in the Brain, and if So, What Are They?

Emerging research in neuroscience has provided compelling evidence that mindfulness practice can lead to tangible changes in the brain, a phenomenon often referred to as neuroplasticity. Neuroplasticity is the brain's ability to reorganize itself by forming new neural connections throughout life. This adaptability is fundamental to learning from experiences and how our behaviors and environment can shape our brain's structure and function. Mindfulness meditation can significantly influence this process by emphasizing sustaining attention to the present moment and fostering openness and curiosity.

Studies using magnetic resonance imaging (MRI) have shown that regular mindfulness meditation can increase the thickness of the prefrontal cortex, a part of the brain associated with higher-order brain functions such as awareness, concentration, and decision-making. This thickening of the cortex mirrors the strengthening of these cognitive abilities and indicates the brain's plasticity in response to mindfulness practice. Similarly, decreased brain cell volume in the amygdala, which is responsible for fear, anxiety, and stress responses, has been observed. These changes suggest that mindfulness meditation could reduce feelings of stress and improve emotional well-being.

Furthermore, mindfulness has been associated with changes in the default mode network (DMN), a brain network implicated in self-referential thoughts and mind-wandering. Studies suggest that mindfulness practice reduces activity in the DMN, which is significantly active during periods of rest and is known to engage in the kind of self-referential thoughts that can lead to anxiety and depression. By reducing activity in this network, individuals may experience fewer negative thoughts about themselves and improved well-being. Additionally, mindfulness meditation has been linked to enhanced connectivity between the DMN and other brain regions responsible for attention and executive control, suggesting an improved ability to switch out of self-referential modes of thinking and engage more effectively with the external world.

The tangible changes in the brain attributed to mindfulness practice highlight its potential as a powerful tool for enhancing cognitive and emotional health. By fostering neuroplastic changes, mindfulness improves current mental health conditions and equips individuals with a resilience that supports long-term well-being. These findings underscore the importance of incorporating mindfulness practices into daily routines for those seeking to harness the benefits of a more flexible and adaptive brain.

Thank You

We are deeply grateful for your time in reading this book. Your dedication to exploring the profound effects of mindfulness on physical and mental health is commendable.

We hope the insights and research shared have inspired you to integrate mindfulness practices into your life, unlocking the potential for enhanced well-being and resilience.

May your mindfulness journey lead to meaningful transformations, empowering you to live a more balanced life. Thank you for allowing us to be a part of your personal and professional growth.